Stay Youthful Forever

Tanushree Podder

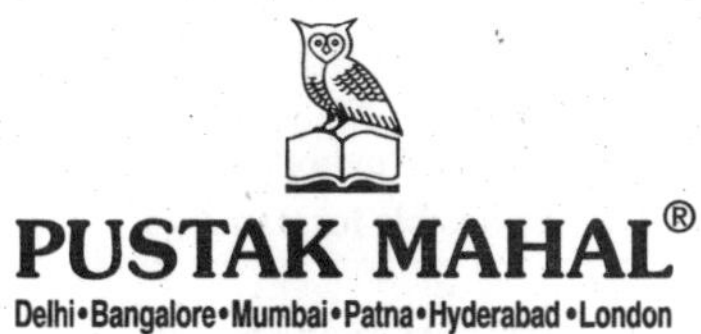

PUSTAK MAHAL®
Delhi • Bangalore • Mumbai • Patna • Hyderabad • London

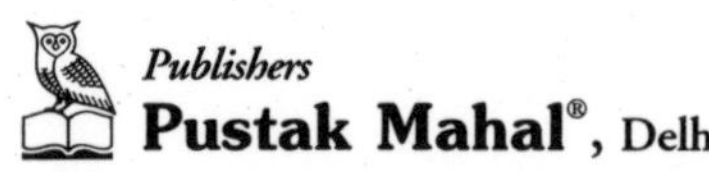

Publishers
Pustak Mahal®, Delhi

J-3/16 , Daryaganj, New Delhi-110002
☎ 23276539, 23272783, 23272784 • *Fax:* 011-23260518
E-mail: info@pustakmahal.com • *Website:* www.pustakmahal.com

London Office
5, Roddell Court, Bath Road, Slough SL3 OQJ, England
E-mail: pustakmahaluk@pustakmahal.com

Sales Centre
10-B, Netaji Subhash Marg, Daryaganj, New Delhi-110002
☎ 23268292, 23268293, 23279900 • *Fax:* 011-23280567
E-mail: rapidexdelhi@indiatimes.com

Branch Offices
Bangalore: ☎ 22234025
E-mail: pmblr@sancharnet.in • pustak@sancharnet.in
Mumbai: ☎ 22010941
E-mail: rapidex@bom5.vsnl.net.in
Patna: ☎ 3294193 • *Telefax:* 0612-2302719
E-mail: rapidexptn@rediffmail.com
Hyderabad: *Telefax:* 040-24737290
E-mail: pustakmahalhyd@yahoo.co.in

ISBN 978-81-223-0751-1

Edition : August 2007

This book was earlier printed under the title
"Youthful Forever"

Printed at : **Unique Colour Carton. New Delhi-110 064**

Dedication

I did not have to spend a single moment thinking about whom I was going to dedicate this book to. It was so very clear; right from the time I conceived the idea about writing this book.

This book is dedicated to my sterling lifemate, Ajoy. Youthful, relaxed and in control, he is the ultimate symbol of fitness. Touchwood!!

PREFACE

Man has always wanted to remain youthful. He has wandered in search of the ultimate panacea to ageing, seeking his immortality and youth. Being youthful is a state of mind. There are hundreds of people who do not look their age and to those hundreds there are thousands who look older than age. It is all to do with the mind-body and spirit connection. With research, it is becoming more and more evident that our bodies are governed and controlled by our mind. In fact, about 85% people residing in the urban areas suffer from ailments that have no organic origin. The amazing impact of our thoughts on our body and health is beyond comprehension.

Why do people age? This is a mystery that is yet to be solved by the scientists. One cannot stop the process of ageing but one can certainly retard it by a considerable extent. It is difficult to put the clock back but holding it is possible. Science has increased the life span of human beings. One look around us will reveal quite a few interesting things. Today, the youth are greying and ageing at a faster rate than people did about a couple of generations back; it is not uncommon to find young men and women with greying hair, aged and unhealthy bodies. The youth today are unhealthier than the earlier generation at their age. In fact, one can still find active sixty or seventy year olds. They are fitter and healthier because of the lifestyle they had observed during their youth. In so many cases, I have found the parents to be fitter than their children.

The present generation has a stress ridden existence, which when combined with unhealthy eating habits, environmental pollution and sedentary habits, can only spell trouble. Considering this, it is not surprising that people are ageing at a faster rate than ever before. What they need to do is to jump off the fast track and decelerate their lives.

What is it that ages one person faster than the other, all things being equal? There are four major factors that can be counted for this malady.

• Wrong diet • Lack of exercise • Stress • Environmental hazards

Many of us look after our cars better than we look after ourselves. We snatch hurried meals, often of 'convenience' foods, sleep fitfully, without being properly relaxed, travel stressfully in crowded buses or trains or drive in traffic choked roads, our lives ruled by the clock. We accept excessive demands from home and work, incessantly neglecting our real needs, but eventually the constant strain of living out of tune with ourselves begins to take its toll. We may become irritable and overtired and fall prey to a host of minor infections, aches and pains. Sadly, however, few of us stop to ask why we are doing all this and still fewer of us recognise our ills as a consequence of our own self-neglect.

To remain youthful and healthy, one does not start at the age of fifty, but it is a gradual process of self-discipline, nurturing healthy habits and a perception of the long time goal. The earlier one begins to maintain healthy habits, the better. I would go to the extent of saying that one should begin with the discipline when one is in the twenties.

We do not think about ageing when we are twenty, it seems so far away. We continue to abuse our body, subjecting it to all kinds of unhealthy treatments of lifestyle. We do not even think about it when we are thirty; ageing still remains a distant problem. We are busy making time for our career and future. It is only when we are in our late thirties rather early forties, I would say, when we start worrying about the ageing process. We begin to worry, not because it is no longer a distant problem, but because the years of neglect begin to take a toll on our health.

It is said that longevity of human beings has increased in the last three decades. Has it really? I think that people lived longer and were healthier, about fifty years back than they are now. Lesser number of people died from coronary attacks and diabetes or cancer than today. The young were strong and youthful unlike the present youth. The major advances in improving life span made by medical science have been a result of decreased infant and child mortality. However, if you remove the child mortality factor from the life expectancy figures, it will be obvious that we are not doing as well as we may have concluded. In fact, the probability of living longer and healthier after the age of forty has remained relatively constant.

In a bid to enjoy our lives, we live in a fast lane that leaves us no time to care for our body. It is like buying a new and flashy car. It runs very well initially and we enjoy the drives, not really bothering about the maintenance part. After all, it is running fine! A few years later, it begins giving us problems. The shine and gloss fade and the mechanical parts start wearing out. We begin getting a little worried but still we do not find the time to give it our attention. Then one fine day, just as we are returning from a party, late at night, our faithful car stops suddenly at a lonely spot. We curse it, kick it and try all stunts but it refuses to budge. The neglect of all the years has taken its toll. We suddenly realise that we should have taken better care of the car, which would have prevented our getting stranded on the roadside.

I have given this analogy to illustrate how our lifestyle influences our body and how we continue to neglect it when we are young. Instead, if we were to pay a little attention to the body in our prime years, it will serve us better in the later years of our life. Looking and feeling youthful is all a part of being aware of the requirements of the body and giving it the due respect.

Caring for the body should begin even as we are in our twenties. It is never too early to start respecting our bodies.

This book, therefore, is aimed at teaching you to be aware of and to honour your own needs, both physically and psychologically, so that you can avoid some of the damages on your health and energy, that twenty-first century living can entail. Heed now to the needs of your body, listen to it and stop abusing it!

–Tanushree Podder

CONTENTS

Section One
A YOUTHFUL BODY

Section Two
YOUTHFUL FOOD

Section Three
YOUTHFUL LIFESTYLE

Section Four
YOUTHFUL SPIRIT

Section One A YOUTHFUL BODY

What really is a youthful body? A youthful body, to some people, would mean having boundless energy, vitality and an irrepressible spirit. To others it would mean having a body that is without any disease and to yet others, it could mean leading a full life without the hassles of being worried about fatigue and tiredness. To me it means having a spring in the walk, a song on the lips and a general feel-good attitude. It also means being strong enough to cope with all kinds of adversities and situational crises.

In fact, all these premises are correct. A youthful body is one, which doesn't lack in energy and vitality and is free of diseases. So what has age got to do with youthfulness of the body? One can remain youthful till a ripe age through fitness and discipline. The process of ageing is not just about the body; it also has a lot to do with one's attitude about life. At the same time, just feeling youthful may not really help unless you are physically fit because when the joints are aching and the energy flagging, youthfulness seems such a far dream. And how does one remain fit and young? That is what we will deal with, in this section.

Chapter 1

YOUTHFUL FITNESS

Being youthful means having a fit body. There cannot be two ways about this. An overweight and unfit person can never remain youthful. We all know the importance of remaining active and energetic. Hundreds of books have been written on this subject. An active life coupled with a regular exercise regimen is the key to a fit body.

The very appearance of a person displays his fitness. A fit person has a glow on the face and a good posture. Fitness of the body can be of two kinds - "Organic fitness", generally pertains to a body free of disease and infirmity; in basic terms it means healthy; while "Dynamic fitness" means endurance, flexibility, and strength of the body.

The awareness about physical fitness has grown in leaps and bounds. If you look out of your window any morning or early evening, you are likely to spot a jogger or a walker. The magazine on your coffee table is likely to have a jogger or a fitness enthusiast on its cover. TV commercials promoting any kind of product, from soap to hardware, may also feature the jogger. Concern over fitness has become a global pre-occupation, and the reasons are not hard to find. The physically fit have stronger hearts and leaner bodies; numerous studies have shown that those who work at becoming fit feel better both physically and mentally.

Amongst the many benefits of a steady and regular exercise regimen, improved efficiency of the heart, lungs and muscles as well as improved posture, rank high. An important aspect of physical fitness is the effect it has on the way we feel about ourselves. A straight back, a spring in the walk and an alert, energetic expression are some of the fallouts of the improved self-esteem that comes along with a fit and energetic body. A fat and unfit person with a slouching posture, slumped shoulders and uncoordinated movements is hardly someone who is going to nurture a high self-esteem.

Fitness has an added advantage because the very approach to life changes, resulting in quality life. It brings with it, an optimistic outlook, energetic view and effervescent mind. A fit person can be spotted from a distance because he stands out in a crowd. Need we say more? The advantages of fitness are not unknown and every human being wants to be fit. But most people are on the lookout for an easy way out. No wonder the markets are flooded with books, newspapers and magazines that carry articles on instant fitness. The truth is that there are no short cuts to fitness; remember the saying – 'no pain, no gain', it is the ultimate truth as far as fitness is concerned. It is a slow and arduous climb, especially if one is obese and unhealthy.

Physical Fitness

Physical fitness is to the human body what fine-tuning is to an engine. It enables us to perform up to our potential. Fitness can be described as a condition that helps us look, feel and do our best. More specifically, it is: "The ability to perform daily tasks vigorously and alertly, with energy left over for enjoying leisure-time activities and meeting emergency demands. It is the ability to endure, to bear up, to withstand stress, to carry on in circumstances where an unfit person could not continue, and is a major basis for good health and well-being."

As you undertake your fitness programme, it's important to remember that fitness is an individual quality that varies from person to person. It is influenced by age, sex, heredity, personal habits, exercise and eating practices. You can't do anything about the first three factors. However, it is within your power to change and improve the others, where needed.

Around the mid-forties the natural ageing process begins to show itself more obviously, especially if you are unfit, overstressed, or overweight. This is a time when many people are actually at their best, emotionally and psychologically, but health risks are increasing.

For example, about one in ten people in their middle age suffer from problems of peptic ulcers or hypertension. The risk of heart disease, another stress related problem, also increases at this time of life. At this point fitness takes on a special meaning because one needs to halt the degeneration of the physical self.

Quite simply, a sedentary lifestyle shortens your life span. In fact, it's twice as likely to kill you as a high cholesterol level. It gives that old saying "use it or lose it", a whole new meaning, don't you think? When you engage in regular physical activity, every cell in your body reaps the benefits. Exercise lowers your heart rate and blood pressure, strengthens your arteries and bones, speeds your reflexes, boosts your brain power, gives you a euphoric feeling of well being and peps up your entire life. Exercise is addictive, it gives a 'high' no drug or drink can beat. And the best part is that the 'high' is totally harmless.

But what does the fitness revolution mean to the older individual who may never have been an athlete and who seldom engages in strenuous physical activity? A study conducted on the attitudes of the older generation towards physical activity and fitness revealed the following facts:

- It is believed that the need for physical activity decreases and may actually disappear as individuals age.
- There is a tendency to exaggerate the risks involved in vigorous physical activity after middle age.
- The benefits of light, occasional activity are highly overrated.
- Older individuals underrate their own abilities and capacities.

The risks of physical activity for the ageing

A sudden run at full tilt to the limit of physical endurance would be a risky endeavour for someone past middle age. But a brisk walk or easy jog until one begins to tire, then slowing to a walk until rested before resuming the faster pace, definitely entails little or no risk.

Leading doctors contend that the risk of dying while exercising is extremely remote. Minimum risk can be realised by beginning an activity programme at a low, easy level and increasing it gradually to a more strenuous level. It is also advisable to have a physical examination before making any major change in the level of physical activity. Any sign of chest pain or unusual dizziness is an indication that the activity should be stopped immediately.

The physical examinations are required more for the sedentary individuals than the ones who are physically active. Studies support the connection between inactivity and heart disease as well as other problems like obesity.

The Overrated Benefits of Light Activity

Though many people, in middle-age bracket, enjoy activity such as golf or gardening, these activities are of little or no benefit to the heart. Strengthening the heart requires an activity that stimulates the pulse rate to at least 100 per minute for those of the age 55, which is repeated three times a week for periods of fifteen minutes or more. Thus, only a quick run to the first tee on the golf course, or vigorous work with a hoe in the garden will cause the heart to reach the minimum rate necessary to achieve some benefit.

Women who think that housework makes them fit and compensates for exercise, are also in for a shock. The benefits of a regular exercise regime, no matter how light, cannot be compensated through daily or routine activities.

Regular Exercise

As far as exercise is concerned, the best phrase to sum up the importance of movement to your body and health is 'Use it or lose it'. Inactivity, a sedentary lifestyle, means that our bodies are steadily deteriorating and various health problems begin taking a toll. Equally important is the fact that exercise keeps stress and tension effects in check. It makes us feel better, too.

The value of exercise is high at all times of life. In childhood it is essential for growing up and developing strong bones and muscles, for adults it is necessary for keeping fit, and for older people exercise is essential in order to reduce problems like osteoporosis and maintain mobility as well as remain independent.

We all know that a healthy diet and adequate exercise are the '*mantra*' to a fit and healthy life. Although many books and magazines are devoted to encouraging us to work on these factors, they provide so much advice and differing theories and methods that it seems difficult to fulfil these aims. The aim here is to provide information on some of the exercises, which are more relevant to keeping the body youthful while being easy to perform.

There are certain golden rules for following an exercise regimen, one of them being that a minimum of 20 minutes of brisk exercise at least three times a week has to be maintained in order to derive any benefit from it. Having activity goals can be very useful, but they should not act as a deterrent to getting started; any amount of exercise is better than none. I would like to emphasise here that sudden, unaccustomed or inappropriate exercise can cause musculo-skeletal problems and people with certain conditions must seek medical advice before undertaking an exercise regimen.

The first advice is to take the kinds of exercise that you enjoy and that you can easily incorporate into your lifestyle. Walking up and down stairs rather than taking the lift can be a simple example of fitting more movement into your life. Weekend walks, gardening, cycling or dancing are some leisure activities that can also help you to get fitter.

If you have not done much exercise for some time, do try to warm up and loosen the body before doing anything more strenuous and don't exercise right after a meal. If you are ill or very tired, then limit the physical exertion.

Benefits of Regular Exercise

Exercises help to work out the muscles, joints, cardiovascular system, etc, so that when the time comes, normal work can be done without much strain, even in old age. A fit old man can run faster and catch a bus leaving an unfit younger person far behind, when the time comes. No wonder many commercials have this theme to promote their health products. Physical exercises help in increasing blood circulation, provide the muscles with oxygen through the blood streams. All this contributes to greater physical endurance and helps to accomplish daily tasks without much fatigue.

Exercises are the main means of burning calories, thereby keeping obesity in check and creating a pleasant feeling of fitness. Even if you may not become conscious of it immediately, exercise brings with it an improvement of posture, appearance and self-image.

Exercises help to keep the internal organs toned up and perform to their optimum; this in turn helps keep illness away.

The long-term benefit of exercise is that the body is not allowed to gain weight and movement is relatively easier compared to an obese person, and the muscles retain the ability to flex more thereby providing more vigour to the body. This, by itself, is enough to generate the feel-good factor.

The hidden benefits of exercising are many, but the main benefit seems to be the ability of the mind to cope up with stress. A fit person laughs more easily and enjoys the very business of living. It is a natural outcome of being fit because it you exercise well, you sleep well, and if you sleep well you remain devoid of stress and fatigue.

Exercise strengthens your heart and trains it to use oxygen more efficiently. As your heart grows stronger, it can pump more blood through your body, which helps your body function. Regular exercise can help keep your arteries more elastic, and build up muscles and bones at the same time. It also keeps you flexible so you can do all the activities you like. Because your muscles need energy to function while exercising, you'll burn calories, which helps you lose weight, lose body fat and gain lean muscles. Exercise can also help speed up you metabolism.

Regular exercise has been shown to decrease the risk of heart disease, the number one killer in today's world. It has also been known to prevent certain cancers, combat obesity, increase flexibility and range of motion, improve your mood and stamina, and give you an injection of overall energy. In fact, aerobic exercise can also improve your mental health and ability to think, as well as perform and be creative. And if you exercise regularly, it serves as a good model for children. They are more likely to make exercise a habit if they see you doing it. Experts report that by increasing your fitness level even by minimal amounts, you are actually adding years to your life, no matter when you start or what you look like.

Today, there is a growing emphasis on looking good, feeling good and living longer. Increasingly, scientific evidence tells us that one of the keys to achieving these ideals is fitness and exercise. But if you spend your days at a sedentary job and pass your evenings as a "couch potato," it may require some determination and commitment to make regular activity a part of your daily routine.

Exercise is not just for Olympic hopefuls or supermodels. In fact, you're never too unfit, too young or too old to get started. Regardless of your age, gender or role in life, you can benefit from regular physical activity. If you're committed, exercise in combination with a sensible diet can help provide an overall sense of well-being and can even help prevent chronic illness, disability and premature death.

'Wow!' what a long list of the benefits of exercise? Does anyone need any more reasons to begin an exercise regimen? I am sure not. Here, in a nutshell, is a quickover of the benefits of exercise for easy assimilation.

Improved Health

- Increased efficiency of heart and lungs
- Reduced cholesterol levels
- Increased muscle strength
- Weight loss

Improved Sense of Well-Being

- More energy
- Less stress
- Improved quality of sleep
- Improved ability to cope with stress
- Increased mental acuity

Improved Appearance

- Weight loss
- Toned muscles
- Improved posture

Enhanced Social Life

- Improved self-image
- Increased opportunities to make new friends
- Increased opportunities to share an activity with friends or family members

Increased Stamina

- Increased productivity
- Increased physical capabilities
- Less frequent injuries
- Improved immunity to minor illnesses

Reduced Risk Factors

- Reduced High blood pressure
- Reduced Cigarette smoking
- Controlled Diabetes
- No Obesity
- Improved Low levels of HDL

Conditions under which one Should Not Exercise

- Moderate to severe coronary heart disease that causes chest pain from inimical activity.
- A recent heart attack. A three-month waiting period is considered standard before moderate; medically supervised exercise programme can begin.
- Severe heart valve defects and heart beat irregularities.
- A greatly enlarged heart and certain type of congenital heart disease.
- Uncontrolled diabetes where your blood sugar levels fluctuate constantly.
- High blood pressure not controlled by medication.
- Any infectious disease during its acute stage.
- If your doctor says you have bone, joint or muscle problems that could be made worse by the proposed physical activity.
- If you have a medical condition or other physical reason, not mentioned here, that might need special attention in an exercise programme, i.e. insulin-dependent diabetes.

Testing for Fitness

Anybody who is about to embark on a training programme for fitness – whether they choose walking, running or any other form of exercise

– should first gauge their fitness carefully. Persons of all age groups can carry out the pulse test, flexibility and abdominal strength tests described below. The walking test is a tougher fitness check based on distance covered when walking briskly.

1. Measure Your Pulse

Whichever exercise form you choose, measuring your pulse rate during activity is a good way of testing fitness. It is especially useful for monitoring your progress in the course of aerobic workouts. You should take your pulse once or twice during activity, using the maximum pulse rate formula described below. Your pulse rate should not rise much above this safe limit, and it should drop down quickly.

If you are going beyond your safe limit, you are doing too much for your present level of fitness. Modify your activity, but do keep exercising regularly. As you get fitter your pulse rate during the exercise will not rise so much, so you'll need to work harder to raise it to the safe limit. If you are not getting near the safe limit then you are not doing enough to stretch yourself.

Maximum Pulse Rate Formula

During vigorous exercise your pulse rate may rise steeply, according to how hard you work and to your level of fitness. The following rough formula gives you the safe limit for your age during vigorous exercise.

From 220 deduct your age, and then reduce this number by one quarter.

For example, if you are 40 years old = (220-40)
= $180 \times 3/4$
= 135

In this case your safe limit during activity is 135.

Recovery Rate

It is important that your pulse rate should drop down quickly after exercise, as shown below. If your pulse stays high you should take it easy. Try a gentler form of exercise, and build up your fitness more gradually.

Pulse Counting

All you need is a watch with which you can count seconds. Hold it in your left hand while with the first two fingers of the right hand, you search for the pulse in your left wrist. You can usually find it a little below the base of the left thumb. (Reverse hands if you are left-handed). Start by counting the number of beats of the pulse per 60 seconds. When you do this easily, you can proceed to a quick assessment, counting for just 10 seconds and multiplying by six.

(**Caution**: Your pulse rate is not the only criterion of safety. If you feel severe pain or dizziness, you should stop your exercise, and rest. If these symptoms continue, seek your doctor's advice.)

2. Check Your Flexibility

To test your flexibility, perform the following exercise.

Sit on the floor with your legs straight out before you and stretch forward to touch your toes. If you can reach them without difficulty there is adequate flexibility of the spine and shoulders. If you only reach the mid-shin area you should take up an exercise type that rates high on flexibility. The Surya-Namaskar is an excellent all round stretching exercise.

3. Testing Abdominal Tone

The abdominal muscles deserve special attention, since chronic weakness here exacerbates many common ailments like backache, etc. To assess your abdominal strength, lie down on the floor and fold your arms across your chest. Then try to raise the upper part of your body without any jerking movements.

Your back should be relaxed, not held stiffly, and your legs should remain on the floor. If you can do this easily, your abdominal muscles are in good shape. If it is a bit of a struggle, or all you can do is lift your head, then you need to develop them.

4. General Fitness Test

The test given here was devised by Dr. Kenneth Cooper, to assess fitness according to the distance covered in 12 minutes when walking fast. It is designed for anyone who is under 35 years of age, or for anyone over that age who has been exercising regularly at least 3 times a week for at least 6 weeks before undertaking the test.

If this excludes you it is safest to categorise yourself as 'poor' or 'very poor'. The ideal fitness programme for anyone who rates fair, poor or very poor is aerobic walking.

Rating	Distance covered in 12 minutes
Excellent	3.2 km
Good	2.4 – 3.2 km
Fair	2.0 – 2.4 km
Poor	1.6 – 2 km
Very poor	1.6 km

Planning a Balanced Exercise Regimen

To achieve complete fitness you should design yourself a varied exercise programme, combining three distinct elements.

Firstly, to stimulate your circulatory and respiratory systems and increase their capacity, you need a form of aerobic exercise. This can be tailored to your fitness level, and should be practised for about 25 minutes every other day–longer if you choose a gentle type of exercise like walking.

Secondly, you need some form of daily stretching and loosening exercise.

And thirdly, you should choose a regular relaxation technique to refresh and restore you.

For instance, your three-point programme could include aerobic walking for stimulating your circulatory and respiratory systems, *Surya Namaskar* for stretching and loosening your muscles and *Shavasana* as a relaxation technique.

The process of warming up, stretching, loosening of the muscles and finally the cooling down after the exercises is very important. Failing to observe these rules can actually land you in deep trouble and muscle injury.

Warm-up / Cool Down

Before you begin bicycling, walking or running, do some deep massage to your whole knee area. That means above and below, front and back of the knee. Then massage your lower back and ankle areas. Begin your workout slowly. Use good posture and technique. As your body warms up, let your pace rise with it. When it seems that you are ready to really pick up your pace, stop and do some stretching. Then get back to the pace you had just before you stopped.

The process of cooling down after the workout is equally important. When you finish your workout, it is the best time for a relaxing set of stretches. Lie down on a padded floor mat and put you legs up against a wall for a few minutes, taking this time to relax and recoup.

Do some gentle stretching on a padded floor mat and if you have the time, a few minutes on a treadmill or exercise bike will help flush the garbage out of your muscles. The basics of warming-up and cooling-down are lifelong rules that will keep you from undue muscle strain. Remember that the heart is a muscle too and that it is protected by this warm-up and cool down rules.

Stretching

Stretching helps lengthen the working areas of the muscle, allowing for greater work capacity. So as long as your flexibility is balanced and you are stretching intelligently, the more flexible you are, the better. The same goes with strength. So long as you have developed strength over a long period of time and have strength in all areas of your body, you can't be too strong. Stretching should be a lifelong habit rather than just something you do in conjunction with a workout.

There are specific stretches for specific activities. Stretching in one muscle has an effect on the muscles around it. So, put some thought into how and why you are stretching. Stretching as it relates to lifestyle will help us retain and increase our range of motion, making us more capable of doing many activities throughout our lives.

Loosening up Exercise

These exercises are very necessary before undertaking the exercises or sport activity, which demand a lot of stress and endurance for prolonged periods.

Head Circling – Stand erect with both feet comfortably apart. Place hands on the hips. Pull down chin and look down, circle or rotate the head in one direction 10 times, and then again 10 times in the opposite direction.

Arm Circling – Stand erect with legs comfortably apart and hands on both sides. Raise the hands from the front upwards, and bring them down to the sides again from the rear without bending the elbows. Do this 10 times in one direction and then in the other direction.

Trunk Twisting – Stand erect with legs comfortably apart and hands at the side. Turn from the trunk upwards to the left and then to the right without lifting the feet off the ground. Repeat the whole exercise 10 times each side.

Knee Clasping – Stand erect with legs comfortably apart and hands to the side. Lift one knee bent to the chest. Clasp the knee with both hands and pull towards the chest with pressure. Repeat this 10 times with each knee.

Toe Touching – Stand erect with legs comfortably apart. Bend forward without bending the legs to touch the toes with the fingers, and then return to upright position again. Repeat this ten times.

Getting Started

Be Committed

You have taken the important first step on the path to physical fitness by seeking information. The next step is to decide that you are going to be physically fit.

The decision to carry out a physical fitness programme cannot be taken lightly. It requires a lifelong commitment of time and effort. Exercise must become one of those things that you do without question, like bathing and brushing your teeth. Unless you are convinced of the benefits of fitness and the risks of unfitness, you will not succeed. Patience is essential. Don't try to do too much too soon and don't quit before you have a chance to experience the rewards of improved fitness. You can't regain in a few days or weeks what you have lost in years of sedentary living, but you can get it back if you persevere. And the prize is worth the price.

The Workout Schedule

How often, how long and how hard you exercise, and what kinds of exercises you do should be determined by what you are trying to accomplish. Your goals, your present fitness level, age, health, skills, interest and convenience are among the factors you should consider. For example, an athlete training for high-level competition would follow a different program than a person whose goals are good health and the ability to meet work and recreational needs.

Your exercise programme should include something from each of the four basic fitness components described above. Each workout should begin with a warm-up and end with a cool-down. As a general rule, space your workouts throughout the week and avoid consecutive days of hard exercise. Here are the amounts of activity necessary for the average, healthy person to maintain a minimum level of overall fitness. Included are some of the popular exercises for each category.

Warm-up – 5-10 minutes of exercises such as walking, slow jogging, knee lifts, arm circles or trunk rotations. Low intensity movements that stimulate movements to be used in the activity can also be included in the warm up.

Muscular strength – a minimum of two 20-minute sessions per week that include exercises for the entire major muscle groups.

Muscular endurance – at least three 30-minute sessions each week that include exercises such as callisthenics, push-ups, sit-ups, pull-ups, and weight training for all the major muscle groups.

Cardio respiratory endurance – Carry out at least three 20-minute bouts of continuous aerobic (activity requiring oxygen) rhythmic exercise each week. Popular aerobic conditioning activities include brisk walking, jogging, swimming, cycling, rope jumping, rowing, cross-country skiing, and some continuous action games like racquetball and handball.

Flexibility – 10-12 minutes of daily stretching exercises performed slowly without a bouncing motion. This can be included after a warm-up or during a cool-down.

Cool down – a minimum of 5-10 minutes of slow walking, low-level exercise, combined with stretching.

Controlling Your Weight

The key to weight control is keeping energy intake (food) and energy output (physical activity) in balance. When you consume only as many calories as your body needs, your weight will usually remain constant. If you take in more calories than your body needs, you will put on excess fat. If you expend more energy than you take in you will burn excess fat. Exercise plays an important role in weight control by increasing energy output, calling on stored calories for extra fuel. Recent studies show that not only does exercise increase metabolism during a workout, but it causes your metabolism to stay increased for a period of time after exercising, allowing you to burn more calories.

How much exercise is needed to make a difference in your weight depends on the amount and type of activity, and on how much you eat. Aerobic exercise burns body fat. A medium-sized adult would have to walk more than 30 miles to burn up 3,500 calories, the equivalent of one pound of fat. Although that may seem like a lot, you don't have to walk the 30 miles all at once.

Walking a mile a day for 30 days will achieve the same result, providing you don't increase your food intake to negate the effects of walking. If you consume 100 calories a day more than your body needs, you will gain approximately 10 pounds in year. You could take that weight off, or keep it off, by doing 30 minutes of moderate exercise daily. The combination of exercise and diet offers the most flexible and effective approach to weight control.

Since muscle tissue weighs more than fat tissue, and exercise develops muscle to a certain degree, your bathroom scale won't necessarily tell you whether or not you are "fat." Well-muscled individuals, with relatively little body fat, invariably are "overweight" according to standard weight charts. If you are doing a regular programme of strength training, your muscles will increase in weight, and possibly your overall weight will increase. Body composition is a better indicator of your condition than body weight.

Lack of physical activity causes muscles to get soft, and if food intake is not decreased, added body weight is almost always fat. Once active people, who continue to eat as they always have after settling into sedentary lifestyles, tend to suffer from "creeping obesity."

Clothing

All exercise clothing should be loose-fitting to permit freedom of movement, and should make the wearer feel comfortable and self-assured. As a general rule, you should wear lighter clothes than temperatures might indicate. Exercise generates great amounts of body heat. Light-colour clothing that reflects the sun's rays is cooler in the summer, and dark clothes are warmer in winter. When the weather is very cold, it's better to wear several layers of light clothing than one or two heavy layers. The extra layers help trap heat, and it's easy to shed one of them if you become too warm.

In cold weather, and in hot, sunny weather, it's a good idea to wear something on your head. Never wear rubberised or plastic clothing. Such garments interfere with the evaporation of perspiration and can cause body temperature to rise to dangerous levels.

The most important item of equipment for the runner is a pair of sturdy, properly fitting running shoes. Training shoes with heavy, cushioned soles and arch supports are preferable to flimsy sneakers and light racing flats.

When to Exercise?

Most people prefer the morning hours for exercise. The hour just before the evening meal is also a popular time for exercise. The late afternoon workout provides a welcome change of pace at the end of the workday and helps dissolve the day's worries and tensions. Another popular time to work out is early morning, before the workday begins. Advocates of the early start say it makes them more alert and energetic on the job.

Among the factors you should consider in developing your workout schedule are personal preference, job and family responsibilities, availability of exercise facilities and weather. It's important to schedule your workouts for a time when there is little chance that you will have to cancel or interrupt them because of other demands on your time. You should not exercise strenuously during extreme hot, humid weather, or within two hours after eating. Heat and/or digestion both make heavy demands on the circulatory system, and in combination with exercise can be an overtaxing double load.

Which Exercises?

This is one of the commonest dilemmas faced by people today. Since there are hundreds of kinds of exercises one doesn't know which one would suit the best or work out for someone. Different magazines, books, television programmes advocate different kinds of workouts. I have myself tried out dozens of things till I realised that each individual has his own body requirements based on his weight, lifestyle, health factors and food habits. What works for A need not work for B. In fact, it can sometimes be quite hazardous to try out some vigorous exercise if one is not very fit.

As one grows older, one has to take into consideration things like muscle injury, and risk factors of a heavy exercise regimen. The tendons and ligaments of an ageing body require sensitive handling so one must avoid rigorous exercising regimens. Even if one were to adopt these regimens, the progress has to be gradual and careful.

Some of the excellent exercise routines I discovered were the traditional kind, which were based on scientific wisdom and knowledge. These have their base on holistic handling of the fitness, which covers mind, body and soul. Whether it is the yoga, Tibetan rites of youth or Makko-ho, they combine an effective end result with easy performance and no risk involvement.

These exercises can be performed by persons of any age right from a child to the elderly. They are very effective in keeping the body fit and elevate the performer to a heightened spiritual level. I would recommend these exercises over any other kind, any day.

Apart from these exercises, I personally swear by the efficacy of walking. It is one of the simplest and pleasurable exercises ever discovered.

■■

Chapter 2

YOUTHFUL EXERCISES

Any thing that is not in use deteriorates, just as a nail rusts. By the same logic, our body also begins to show signs of rusting if we do not use it well. In this case, using the body is just another way ofsaying that a body needs exercise. As we have already seen, exercise is the key to fitness and youthfulness. There are hundreds of exercises devised for the purpose of keeping the body fit and most of them are quite effective, too. I came across this set of exercises that are especiallygeared for the purpose of retaining youthfulness. These exercises are not too difficult to perform once the body has loosened up and the muscles are toned.

1. Tibetian Rites of Youth

From ancient times, the Tibetan Lamas have been performing some exercises, which are almost like rituals for them. Have you ever wondered why the monks remain youthful looking and have an enviable longevity of life? Well, the secret for their youthful looks is the set of exercises they perform, unfailingly and with the same devotion they observe for the other religious rites. The principles, on which the exercises are centred, are the seven 'Chakras' or the 'Vortexes'. Most Asians have believed that these Chakras are the energy centres and are connected with the functioning of the endocrine glands. Anyone can perform this set of five exercises or rites, which are very simple.

Firstly, one must understand what is the significance of each chakra and what they represent.

The Seven Chakras are:

1. *Muladhara*, the base chakra, seat of the will to live, corresponds to the sacral plexus and to the adrenals, which rouse the body to action.
2. *Swadhishthana,* corresponds to the prostatic plexus, and the gonads which rule our sexual nature and activity.

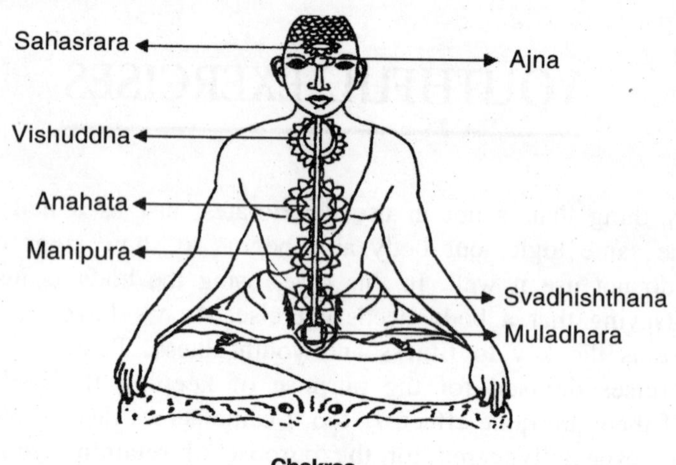

Chakras

3. *Manipura* stores *prana*, and corresponds to the solar plexus, and to the pancreas, which regulates blood sugar, the body's fuel.
4. *Anahata*, the heart chakra, corresponds to the cardiac plexus and the thymus, a vital part of the immune system.
5. *Vishuddha*, the throat chakra, corresponds to the laryngeal plexus and to the thyroid, which governs the body's metabolic rate.
6. *Ajna*, the brow chakra, corresponds to the cavernous plexus and the pituitary, the master gland, which rules the endocrine system.
7. *Sahasrara*, the crown chakra, seat of the highest consciousness, corresponds to the pineal, a mysterious gland thought to govern sleeping and waking.

Rite No 1 – It is a very simple exercise. Stand erect with your arms out stretched, palms facing the floor. Now spin around till you are a bit dizzy. It is important that you turn from left to right. To get it right, place a clock on the floor; face up, in front of you. Turn in the same direction as the clock arms. Spin slowly six times to start with. If you feel dizzy, sit down and relax for some time. Gradually increase the number of turns till you feel slightly dizzy. A dozen times is good enough as the vortexes get excited and the aim is achieved.

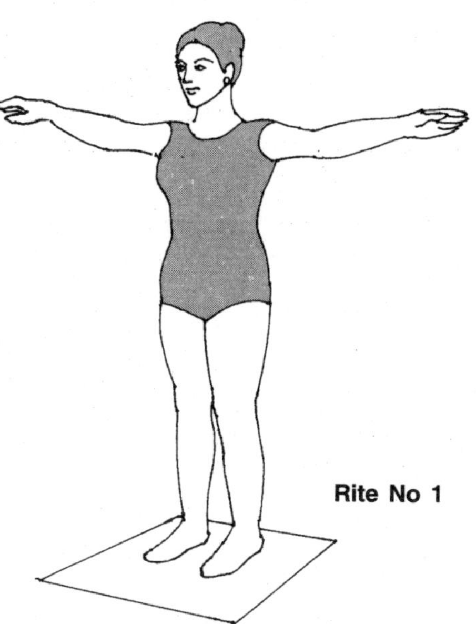

Rite No 1

Rite No 2 – This exercise further excites the vortexes and is comparatively simpler than the first. Lie flat on the back on the floor, which can be covered, with a rug or a carpet to insulate the body and provide a cushion. Keep the arms by the side. Now raise the head and the legs together slowly. Tuck the chin against the chest, and raise the legs, without bending the knees, to a vertical position. Return the head and the legs to the original position slowly and relax. If the legs tend to bend, try to keep them as straight as possible. Breathe in as you raise your head and legs and breathe out as you lower them.

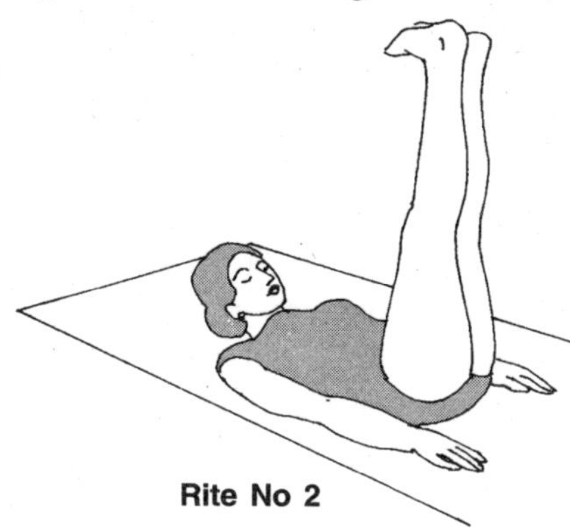

Rite No 2

Rite No 3 – Rite no 3 should be done immediately after Rite no 2. Kneel on the floor with the body erect and the hands placed against the thigh muscle, by the side. First bend the neck forward, tucking the

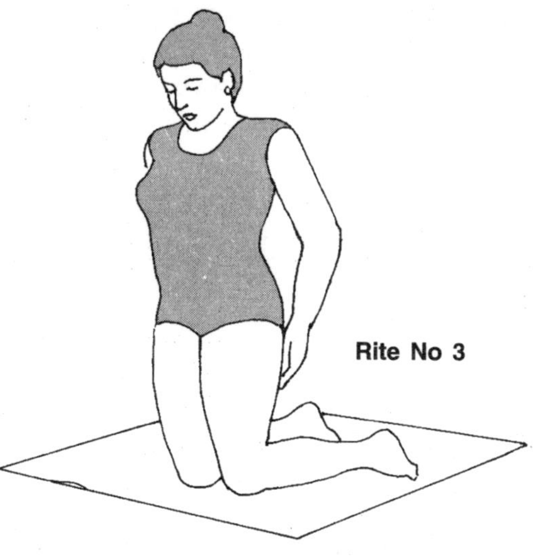

Rite No 3

chin against the chest. Then throw the head and neck back as far as they can go, and at the same time bend backwards, arching the spine. Hold the thighs for support with your hands as you bend backwards. Breathe in as you bend backwards and breathe out as you return to the upright position. Keeping the eyes closed during the exercise avoids distraction.

Rite No 4 – Sit down on the floor with the legs stretched in front of you along the ground, approximately a foot apart. With the trunk of the body erect, place the palms along the body on the floor. First tuck the chin forward against the chest, and then bend backwards. At the same time, taking the weight on the arms raise the body, keeping the arms straight. The body should be in a straight line along with the thighs, parallel to the ground. Repeat this exercise a couple of times, keeping in mind that systematic breathing plays a major role.

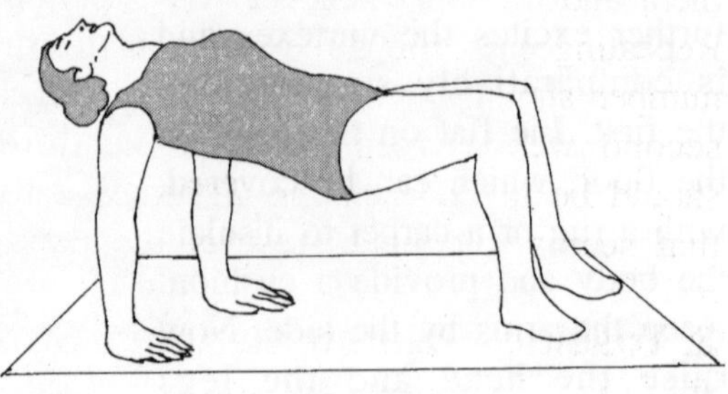

Rite No 4

Rite No 5 – Lie flat on the floor with your face down. Place the palms flat on the floor by the side of the chest. The toes should be flexed on the floor. Look up and raise the chest so that the body arches and the weight of the body is on the toes and palms. Next, bend your head down and raise the hips so that the body forms an inverted " V ". Do this rite slowly, breathing in as you raise the body, and out as you lower it.

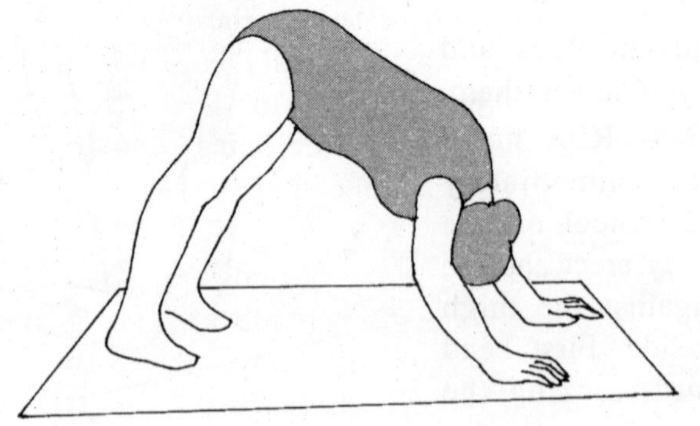

Rite No 5

The Frequency and Duration

The rites should be performed only once a day, and the best time to perform these rites is the early hours in the morning. One can do them at night also. As regards the number of times, one should do the exercises as many times as possible but remember not to overdo them and to stop whenever you experience any feelings of discomfort. Repeating each rite three times in the first week is good enough. The number should be increased by two each week, i.e. five times in the second week, seven times in the third week and so on. The aim should be to do each rite 21 times daily at the end of ten weeks. If that seems too much, restrict the numbers to your comfort-level.

2. Yoseido–Shiatsu Meridian Stretching Exercises

Yoseido is a word with three characters.

Yo – means nourishing, feeding or making something grow.

Sei – means birth - the physiological aspect of a person's existence or simply 'life form'.

Do – means the way, or attaining one's ideal place or spiritual contentment.

The combination of the three words together mean: harmonising one's existing life-form by following the way (the encounter between Heaven and Earth).

Practicing the stretching postures for the eight meridians encourages full health and a lively balance of the energies in our body. They can be used to treat physical ailments by reactivating the flow of vital energy through the body.

They also have a role to play in preventive treatment by ensuring that blocked energy is dislodged, protecting the body from imbalances and stagnation. The exercises are especially beneficial to those with sleeping problems, those with cold hands or feet and those suffering from stress or fatigue. If the exercises are being used for maintenance rather than for specific treatment, then they should be taken in their proper sequence.

The most important posture is for the governing vessel. It is easy to do, and one can quickly experience the effects. If you are not used to exercise and have a very stiff body, start with this exercise alone. It is advisable to do these exercises every morning as well as every evening before going to bed. The spirit of concentration is important. Morning exercise allow us to draw on the rising energy of nature, while evening exercise provides an opportunity to rid our bodies of the tiredness and bad or used energy accumulated during the course of the day. The exercises should not be done after a meal, an operation, or with a fever.

While exercising, it is important to remember that the stretch is made with an inhalation, and that one breathes out slowly after the maximum extension. Breathing out is a vital part of these exercises, because unless we are able to exhale in an even and relaxed way, the next inhalation becomes tight, and then instead of letting the energy flow smoothly into the meridians, we tend to halt the flow of this energy with tense and stumbling breathing. Of course one must not forget someone who is not well and lacks energy will have an entirely different approach to the stretching exercises than someone who is healthy. Either way, it is best to start with the governing vessel and the conception vessel and then go on to the other meridians.

Fortunately each meridian has an important point, which regulates the entire flow of the meridian. So we can start off by pressing these eight points. The regulator point for each of the meridians is as follows:

- Governing vessel: Small intestine point – *"Gokei"*
- Conception vessel: Lung point – *"Reketsu"*
- Yang ankle vessel: Bladder point – *"Shinmiyaku"*
- Yin ankle vessel: Kidney point – *"Shiyokai"*
- Belt vessel: Kidney point – *"Rinkuyu"*
- Through-going vessel: Spleen-pancreas point – *"Koson"*
- Yang linking vessel: Spleen-pancreas point – *"Gaikan"*
- Yin linking vessel: Heart constrictor point – *"Naikan"*

All these points are located near the ankle or close to the wrist - parts of the body which are always in motion and areas where lots of ligaments and tendons are concentrated.

We could say that we walk, jump or run fast because we have solid, strong and supple ankles. Without this movement in the ankle we would be slow and awkward. Our body is constructed to move around using full movement of the muscles in our legs and arms. When we use these muscles with the help of the joints (knee, ankle, elbow, and wrist) we circulate the energy of our internal organs. Arm movements enhance the circulation of lungs and heart, and the movement of legs can activate internal organs such as the small and large intestines.

As we grow old the upper part of our body starts to degenerate first. This manifests itself in grey hair, loss of hair, loss of memory, wrinkles on the face, and weakening of the teeth. In the end we can become immobile because the leg muscles have no strength to hold us straight and let us move. When we become bed ridden, our internal organs start to stagnate, and stop functioning. As long as we can walk, we can keep the organs intact and sustain the minimum vitality of life force.

In China, many elderly people practice the Tai Chi Chuan in public spaces, which keeps them healthy by circulating energy through the entire body. People who are physically disabled or have a rigid constitution can also use the regulating points of the eight meridians.

It is important to acquire the habit of pressing the regulating points daily so that as time goes by one starts to feel more relaxed and notices the benefits of stretching the body. As we know, if the muscles are not regularly stretched and exercised they tighten up, eventually becoming impossible to move. In the case of a broken anklebone plaster is applied to hold the ankle tight during the mending of the fracture. But if these points are pressed right after the accident the healing power can be accelerated.

There is no fixed order for these postures. One can start anywhere. But to strengthen the immune system it is particularly advisable to follow the order given below:

1. Governing Vessel Exercise

- Lying on your back, take hold of the soles of your feet, as illustrated and gently rock on your back, letting your spine roll against the floor.
- It is important to keep your neck soft and long, and not let your chin stick out. All the effort comes from the lower abdomen.

- The movement can start from the coccyx and go up to the first dorsal, avoiding the cervicals of the neck because they are much more delicate.
- Breathe normally during this exercise.

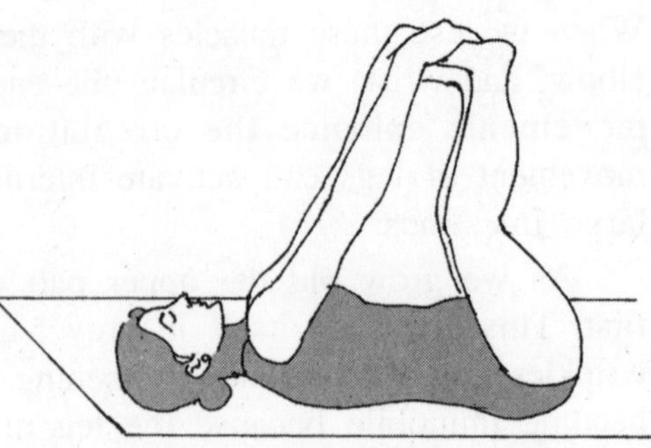
Governing vessel exercise

2. Conception Vessel Exercise

- Lie on your stomach and take hold of your feet, rolling forwards and backwards gently on your stomach, rocking along the centre, and breathing normally.

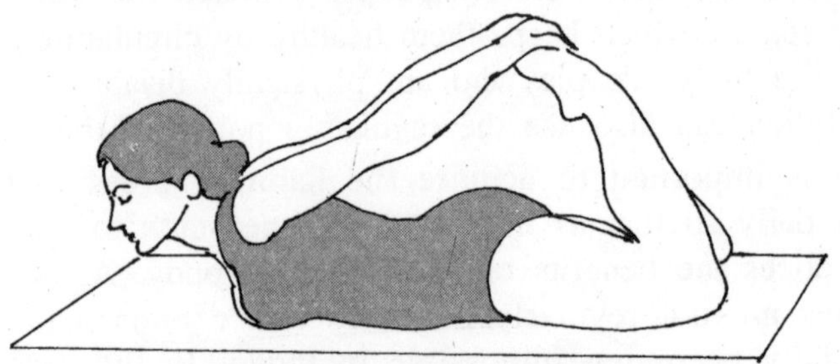
Conception vessel exercise

- If you can't reach your feet with your hands, then imagine you are holding them.
- The aim of the exercise is not to attain a perfect position, but to visualise the posture and follow its possibilities for movement.
- Women should avoid this exercise during a menstrual period, and those with back troubles should not do it until they are feeling better. It does pull on the back.

3. Yang Ankle Vessel Exercise

- Hold the big toe with the thumb and first fingers of the corresponding hand.
- Lift one leg and stretch it towards the outside, and follow it with your eyes, keeping the other leg firmly on the ground.

- Inhale as you lengthen your leg and exhale as you return your leg to the centre.
- Then repeat with the other leg.

4. Yin Ankle Vessel Exercise

- Sit in the Seiza position, as shown, with one leg bent back and close to your body, along the thigh.
- Take hold of the other foot with both hands and lift it up, keeping the leg straight.
- Inhale as you draw it towards your chest.
- Repeat five or six times and then do the same with the other leg.

5. Through Going Vessel Exercise

- Sitting, place one foot on the thigh of the other leg, and stretch forward to hold the other, extended foot with both hands.
- With an inhalation, and the back held straight, draw your body closer to the extended foot.

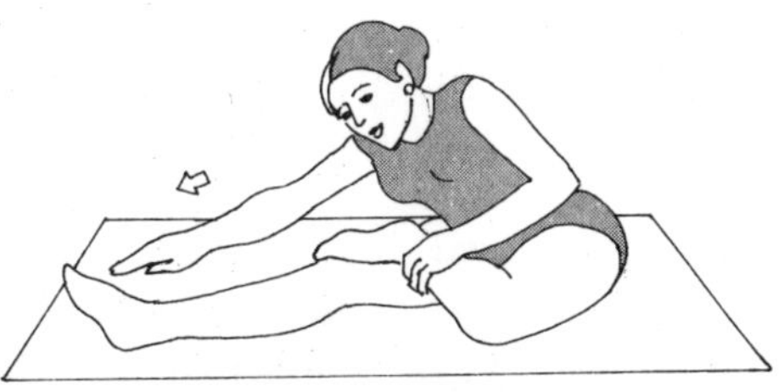

Through-going vessel exercise

- Repeat this exercise five or six times on both legs.

6. Belt Vessel Exercise

- Sit with your legs wide, and place one hand on your hip and the other fairly high along your rib cage.
- With an inhalation lean towards the side where you are holding the hip.
- Repeat the exercise five or six times on each side, and then hold your hands on both hips and make circles with your body from the base of your spine, thirty times in each direction.

7. Yang Linking Vessel Exercise

- Open your legs as wide as you can.
- Place your hands on the floor in front of you.

- Slide your hands slowly forward and with a straight back, let your body go forward. Inhale as you go towards the floor.
- You should stop when you feel it interferes with your breathing.

8. Yin Linking Vessel Exercise

- Sitting, fold your right foot onto the top of the left thigh, holding the foot in place with your right hand stretched across your back.
- Reach forward, keeping the spine straight, and with your left hand take hold of your left foot with your thumb and fingers.
- This exercise is quite difficult but what is important is that you feel as much movements of energy as you can, as you do this.
- If you are very stiff, don't be discouraged, but breathe gently and rhythmically and do what you can.
- Let your imagination recreate the movement, and your body will follow.
- Repeat five or six times for each side.

3. Yoga

Yoga is viewed as many things by different people. The average person thinks yoga is just stretching exercises for bad backs, stress and tension. Yoga is much more. The exercises or *'asanas'* are many and varied, as are the tasks, which they can accomplish. Some of the exercises help to make the body stronger, more flexible and healthier. Others reduce stress and tension and help you to better cope with the trials of everyday life.

Developing your intuition and clear insight is the purpose of other yoga exercises. The underlying purpose of all of the yoga tools is spiritual evolution, the lifting of our consciousness from a mundane, worldly level to an awareness and sensitivity for all creation. Yoga benefits your whole body. Through a systematic set of stretching and strengthening exercises you can stretch and strengthen all of your major muscles groups and develop muscle tone and flexibility. The strengthening of the muscles around the spine is particularly important for keeping the spine in proper alignment and having a healthy, strong spine.

Yoga exercises improve your cardio-vascular system by a strengthening and stretching of the heart muscles and making the arteries and veins more elastic. This elasticity allows the vascular walls to expand and carry more volume of blood to get to the part of the body where it is needed without having to increase the blood pressure. By bending and twisting the body in a myriad of ways, your internal organs get massaged which increases their circulation bringing with the extra blood supply more oxygen and nutrients and taking away with the venous blood flow more toxins and waste material. Similarly, through the bending, twisting, and stretching, you enhance the function of your lymphatic system.

Some yoga exercises improve your eyes, making the eyes healthier, and even help to tone the muscles behind the eyes, which control the shape of the eyes and affect your vision. Through regular practice of yoga postures, your body will regain some of its youth and vigour, making you feel and look younger. You will have more energy and endurance.

Yogic exercises offer a variety of tools for a variety of needs. If you are interested in the just the physical, the mental, the spiritual or all three, yoga works. Yoga is a very effective way of getting fit and healthy, and remaining so. It has its origin in India. The word Yoga means 'communication'. Yoga is pragmatic science, which has been evolved the years and deals with physical, moral, mental and spiritual well-being. There are eight limbs of Yoga as given out by Patanjali in about 200 B.C. These are as follows :

Yama	–	Moral Commandments.
Niyama	–	Purification through discipline.
Pranayama	–	Rhythmic control of the breath.
Asanas	–	Postures, which keep the body healthy and strong.
Pratyahara	–	Freeing the mind from the senses.
Dharana	–	Concentration.
Dhyana	–	Meditation.
Samadhi	–	A state of super consciousness brought about by deep meditation.

The first two control passion and emotion. Pranayama and Pratyahara are known as the inner quest. The last two allow the yogi to realise his 'self'. The relaxation and physical benefits achieved from practising even just once a week are sufficient reward for many beginners and quickly become apparent.

Fitness through Yoga

Stress, fatigue, depression, obesity and heart troubles are some of the most common offshoots of modern lifestyles. India had an answer to the disorders riddling both the mind and the body thousands of years ago in the form of Yoga. So, yoga is a sure fire way to maintain a high level of fitness in the modern day.

Benefits of Yoga

- Regular practice of yoga strengthens the muscles. Yoga controls cholesterol level, reduces weight, keeps your blood pressure under check and generally improves the functioning of the heart.
- Exercises like *Surya Namaskar* improve the capacity of the lungs and oxygenate the blood.
- Stretching and bending during the *asanas* helps in removing hypertension and ensures better functioning of the nervous system.
- Yoga reduces the process of cell deterioration and delays the ageing process.

Surya Namaskar

Although yoga is a vast subject which works both for mental and physical fitness, if you are targeting physical fitness and do not have the time for a range of *asanas, Surya Namaskar* is the regimen for you.

Surya Namaskar or Salutations to the Sun God is a series of 12 postures that can be performed as one complete exercise. The 'surya namaskar' is one of the most comprehensive and basic yogasanas and can be performed every morning or evening or at any convenient time of the day. Surya Namaskar is a warming-up, body toning exercise which energises the body and is also an excellent breath control exercise. All movements should be relaxed and rhythmical and should be practised at least for five minutes every day, to achieve the best results. Here are the 12 postures of Surya Namaskar:

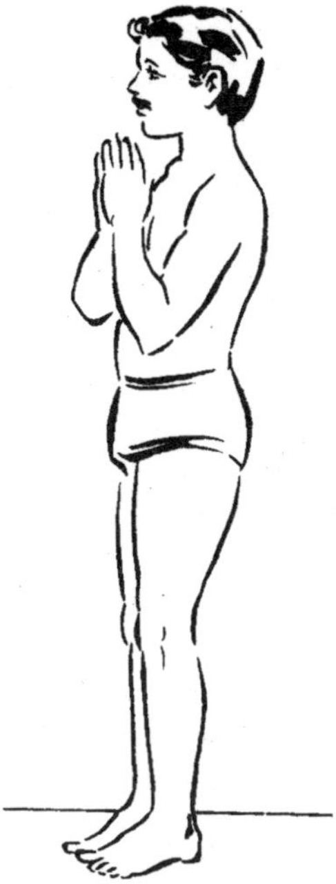

1. ***Namaskarasana***-Stand erect facing the sun, with your palms pressed together against the chest in the namaskar posture. The elbows should be level with the shoulders, and the feet close together. Breathe deeply and relax. This posture is good for the stomach muscles.
2. ***Urdhva Namaskarasana***-Inhale deeply, and raise your arms high above your head, with palms still together and eyes following the hands. Bend your body backwards from the waist, slowly. This asana stretches the front of your body, relaxes muscles, and improves circulation.
3. ***Uttanasana***-Exhale slowly, bend your body forward from the waist, and bring your hands down to the ground in a wide arc. Your head should touch the knees. With practice, you should be able to rest your palms fully on the ground. This asana helps in stretching the back, shoulders and hamstrings.
4. ***Ekapaada Prasaranaasana***-While inhaling, gradually lower the body, raise the head, and move the right leg far back in a wide arc. At the end, the right foot and knee touch the ground, while the left foot remains between the hands. This movement exercises the chest, lower back and legs.
5. ***Dwipaada Prasaranaasana***-As you exhale, extend the left foot and place it next to the right foot. Keep your arms and body straight, and your eyes looking ahead. In this position, you are resting on your hands and toes.
6. ***Bhujangasana***-While inhaling, slowly lower your hips till they are just above the ground. Bend your head and torso as far back as possible. This posture is very good for the spine.

7. ***Ashtaanga Namaskarasana***-While exhaling, slowly lower your body until only the feet, knees, hands, chest and forehead touch the ground. Maintain the posture for a few seconds. Exercises the shoulders, back and chest.

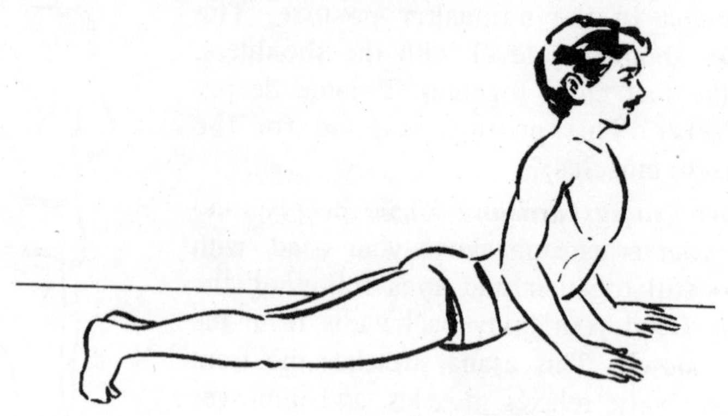

8. ***Bhujangasana***-This is similar to the position in step 6. While inhaling, with hands and feet on the ground, pull your body forward and bend it as far back as you can. Exercises the shoulders, lower back, abdomen and hands.
9. ***Adhomukha Shvaanasana***-As you exhale, curve your body away from the ground. Keep your arms straight, shoulders back, raise your back and hips, and bend your head towards your chest. Exercise the neck, back, hips and legs.
10. ***Ekapaada Prasaranaasana***-While inhaling, return to the position in step 4. Bring your left leg forward and place it between the hands. In the final pose, your right leg is stretched back, and the head is high.
11. ***Uttanasana***-This is the same as the position in step 3. Exhale, and bring the right leg next to the left leg while raising the body. The head touches the knees.
12. ***Back to Namaskarasana***-As you inhale, raise the arms over your head and bend backwards in a repeat of step 2. After that, return to the position in step 1.

Note: Do the exercise in a well-ventilated area, wearing minimal clothing. There are 12 positions in Surya Namaskar, and you should always go through the entire cycle. However, you can take some rest in between exercises. Ensure that your breathing is correct. Much of the benefit of Surya Namaskar is lost if you do not breathe in and out as recommended.

4. Walking

Walking is one of the best exercises I have come across. It rejuvenates, refreshes and brings a sense of euphoria along with the other physical benefits that come with any kind of exercise. All one needs is a good pair of shoes, an open area and a song on the lips.

Walking is an effective, low-impact activity, which is easy on the feet, knees and ankles. This is especially true for people who have joint problems. It is one of the few exercises that a person can continue up to a ripe old age without experiencing any adverse kind of effects.

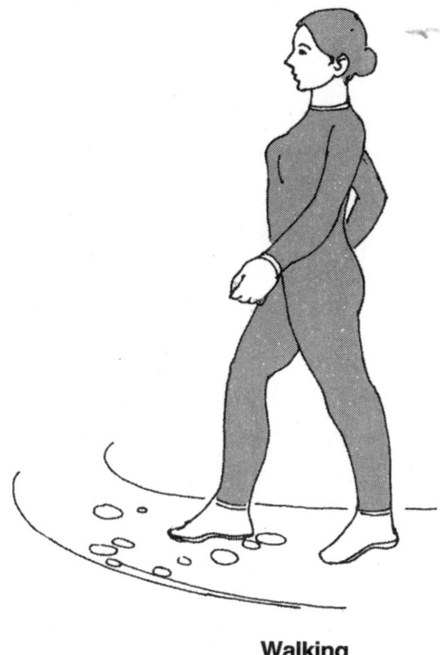

Walking

There are no right and wrong ways of walking. If you are looking for health and fitness, keep pounding the pavements every day of the week for at least 30 minutes. The only factor against walking is the fact that it takes a long time for any kind of visible effect. If you are looking for a quick loss of weight, forget walking and take to some other form of aggressive exercising. But if keeping yourself in a fit form is your goal, welcome to the world of walkers!

For a good aerobic workout, walk tall with your chest out and look straight directing all the motion forward. The arms should be bent at the waist level and not clenched into a tight fist; it should be loosely cupped. The movement of the arms should be to the side of the body, back and forth, and not side to side across the chest. The legs should move in two parallel lines. The body should be relaxed and the stride should be neither too long nor too short but just that comes naturally. No effort should be made to increase or decrease the stride.

Walking can be for different purpose, depending on the speed, purpose and technique. A stroll or leisure walking is slow walking, but at this level it can serve as useful exercise if done for a long time. Fitness walking is at a slightly faster speed and the body begins to sweat. Fitness walking should not be interrupted or halted but should be continuous. Hiking is walking for pleasure and sight seeing. Speed depends on the type of terrain, fitness levels and the weight being carried. Race walking is a sport and governed by a set of rules, which are not discussed here.

Walking can start any time, but not so with running. Jogging or slow running should be combined with walking to start with. Gradually the time devoted to walking should be gradually reduced. Cramps affect the body if one starts running after a long gap or without doing the warming up exercises. Cramps go away as naturally as they come, and if they do not, they are a cause for concern and a doctor should be consulted. Most people take an upward jump while running, this has to change and a forward push is required to be taken.

Benefits of Walking

- **Walking improves circulation** – brisk walking works the heart and speeds up blood circulation along with an increased oxygen intake. Brisk walking affects the human capillary system; this in turn has a chain reaction in revving up the blood circulation and exercising the heart muscles.
- **It clears the mind and has an uplifting effect on mood** – a good walk has an uplifting effect on our mood due to the release of endorphins, which are known mood elevators. The increased supply of oxygen that walking brings, clears the brain and makes it function better.
- **It cuts fatigue and reduces backaches** – walking makes the muscles loosen up and stretches them, too. This results in more mobility and flexibility, which in turn prevents fatigue

from affecting in the muscles. It stretches the spine, thus reducing the incidence of lower backaches.

Let's Start Walking

Thought you mastered walking at age one? Well, think again. Fitness walking isn't an afternoon stroll. I would say that you need to stride rather than walk, to derive the maximum physical benefit. Striding is an easy walking programme that's guaranteed to help you get fit, toned, and on track with a cardiovascular workout.

This training programme will start you off and have you charging full-speed ahead in just seven weeks. Remember, take it slow, and be sensitive to your body. Don't push yourself on days when your tolerance is low, or if you feel the feet need to rest. Drink plenty of water, get lots of sleep, and don't forget to stretch after each walk to keep you in balance.

Walking Schedule

Week 1: This week hit the pavement for 10 minutes on three days. Watch your form as you walk!

Week 2: This week notch up your walking programme to 15 minutes on four days. Try the forward bend each day before you head out!

Week 3: This week log in 20 minutes of aerobic walking on four days. For maximum benefits, use a heart rate monitor and aim for your target heart rate (THR)!

Week 4: Crank up your walking routine an extra notch, to 25 minutes and extend it to five days. Buy yourself a new pair of socks to celebrate!

Week 5: This week hold the line at five days, but add another five minutes to your programme. If you're feeling ambitious, work on your upper body on one of your free days!

Week 6: Maintain your five-day, 30-minute programme. Treat yourself to some soothing lotion. Massage your feet, using firm, circular motions, after your walks.

Week 7: Great going, now just keep walking!

Aerobic Walking

The following programme devised by Dr.Kenneth Cooper, is designed for a low level of fitness. It is a progressive 16-week programme that entails taking 5 walks a week, gradually increasing your time and the distance you cover. All you need is a stopwatch, comfortable and loose clothes and sensible low-heeled walking shoes.

Weeks	Distance covered in each of 5 walks	Time
1	1 mile (1.6 km)	15 minutes
2	1 mile (1.6 km)	14 minutes
3	1 mile (1.6 km)	13 min 45 seconds
4	1½ miles (2.4 km)	21 min 30 seconds
5	1½ miles (2.4 km)	21 min 30 seconds
6	1½ miles (2.4 km)	21 min 30 seconds
7	2 miles (3.2 km)	28 minutes
8	2 miles (3.2 km)	27 min 45 seconds
9	2 miles (3.2 km)	27 min 30 seconds
10	2 miles (3.2 km)	27 min 30 seconds
11	2½ miles (4 km)	35 minutes
12	2½ miles (4 km)	34 min 30 seconds
13	3 miles (4.8 km)	42 minutes
14	3 miles (4.8 km)	42 minutes
15	3 miles (4.8 km)	42 minutes
16	4 miles (6.4 km)	56 minutes

Walking Basics

Stand up straight – Look directly ahead. Imagine that a string is attached to the top of your head and is lifting you from the ground. Keep your shoulders back and relaxed, chest lifted, and tailbone pointing down to the ground.

Relieve the stress points – Relax your shoulders and shake out any tension from your arms and wrists. Bend your arms at the elbow about 83 degrees. Wiggle your fingers and then hold your hands in loose balls (pretend you're clasping a jumbo-size magic marker against your palms). Swing your arms naturally as you walk, but try not to let your hands extend above your chest.

Keep your steps short and fast – The faster you move, the better your cardiovascular workout. Keep an even stride and maintain a steady pace.

Heel-to-toe motion – As you walk, your heel should be the first part of your foot to hit the ground. Roll through the ball of the foot and push off with your toes. This motion reduces the risk of shin splints and tendon pulls.

Care of the Foot

Feet play the most important part in your walking regimen. If they are not cared for, they are not likely to cooperate with you and your fitness programme will end even before it has begun. Most of us are very careless towards foot-health. We often tend to neglect the feet till they really begin to hurt.

When you begin your walking schedule remember to checkout the following aspects.

Blisters – blisters are caused when there is friction against the skin. Friction can be due to the friction between the ground and the foot (if not wearing any foot wear), and between the shoes and the feet. The shoes must fit properly when worn with the socks. Socks act as cushions, especially those made of cotton-acrylic. The socks should be clean and worn dry, on dry feet. Small blisters must be covered with sterile gauze pad. In case of a big blister, puncture it with a sterile needle and clean with antiseptic. Never peal off the skin over a blister.

Calluses and Corns – These do not hurt, however, hard and big ones can be painful under pressure. Rubbing corns with pumice stone after a bath helps. A doctor can cut or file the area. Applying body lotion can soften the area around a callus. Proper fitting shoes, corrected with pad or inserts can avoid callus and make running a pleasure.

Bunions – Bunions are painful swelling on the first joint of the big toe and these are usually hereditary. During walking or running they can get worse and very painful. Small swellings are generally overcome by wearing shoes that are wide in the front and with adequate cushioning. Surgery is recommended only if the bunion becomes painful.

Nails – Nail of the foot should be kept short and at no time should push against the front of the shoe. Nails rubbing against the shoe while running can be painful, the rubbing first occurs with the big toe. Care must be taken to cut the nails across so that they do not become ingrown.

Athlete's Foot – It is a fungal growth on the feet. These occur when hygiene is lax and proper care is not taken of the feet. Shoes should be such that the foot is able to breathe. The shoes should be aired and kept in the sun if possible. Wear shoes dry and spray with anti-fungal powder if the foot is affected. The area between the toes is most prone. In case of persistent problem consult a dermatologist.

Cramps – They are common problems. Simple cramps come and go easily. To avoid cramps, a little workout is necessary before any exercise. Massaging the feet after a workout helps to ease the muscles and prevent stiffness. If there is redness, swelling and pain, it is best to consult a doctor.

The bad news is that if your feet hurt, you're not going to enjoy your walk. The good news is that some common foot problems are fairly easy to treat and easier still to avoid.

Precautions

- Pounding usually causes aching arches when you walk. The first thing you need to do is check your form. Are you landing on your heel and pushing off with your toes? If the problem persists, arch supports might help; if that doesn't work, consult a sports doctor.

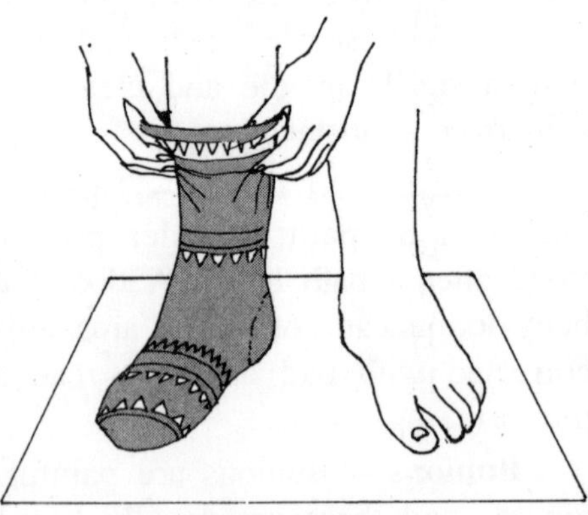

Precautions

- Corns and calluses are painful, and the more you ignore them, the worse they get. Check your shoes to make sure you've got a comfortable fit. And toss thin socks:

You need to have a nice cushion between your feet and inside your shoes.

- Blackened toenails are common and painful, and are caused when your big toe hits the front of your shoe. Keep your toenails neatly trimmed and filed. Check your shoe size and wear double socks on the smaller foot if the shoe is too loose. Most people have one foot that's larger than the other. Always buy your walking shoes for the larger foot.

Foot stretch

Here are two tension-relieving foot stretches that feel great. Remove your shoes and socks before starting these stretches.

- *Stretch 1:* Stand up straight, with your shoulders relaxed down. Hold your abdominal firm to support your back and keep your pelvis in a neutral position (That's when your lower back has a natural curve but not too overarched). Your feet should be hip-width apart. Place your hands on your waist. Slightly bend your knees. Shift your weight back onto your heels and lift your toes off the ground. Flex the front of your feet. Spread your toes as wide as you can. Hold the stretch for the count of five and don't forget to breathe. This will feel terrific before you head out and later when you return home.

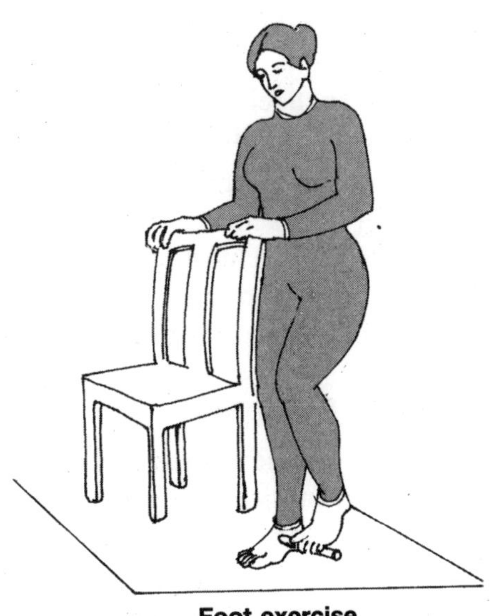

Foot exercise

- *Stretch 2:* Find a comfortable chair and practise picking up magic markers with your toes. Give your toes a nice press, grip the marker, lift your foot five to six inches off the ground, and then set it down. Do this exercise six times, alternating your feet.

■ ■

Chapter 3

YOUTHFUL POSTURE

There is nothing more ageing than a wrong posture. A person with youthful stance looks young and energetic whereas a person (even if he is young) with a stoop, hunch or sloping shoulders presents an ageing look.

This is not the only reason why a person should pay attention to his posture. Ninety percent people, by the time they are 35, complain of backaches and the most common cause of a backache is usually a bad posture. With the growing number of slipped disc cases, spinal and back problems, it becomes doubly important to ensure that good posture becomes a part of one's life.

What is Posture?

Dictionary defines posture as the position of a person's body and the way a person sits or stands. It is judged to be good, normal or bad by the position of the head, chest, trunk, pelvis, knees and feet.

Posture can be a guide to the way people feel. If they are tired, their posture may be poorer than usual. Posture can also reflect mental attitude. Changes in posture may affect a person's appearance, gait, and personality. Good posture gives an impression of poise and self-confidence. It allows the body to function at its best. The best posture is always moving because holding a single position for a long time affects the circulation and respiration. Physical training, learning about body functions, and learning to relax, all aid in posture improvement.

Bad posture can cause many health problems like an aching back, a strained neck, rigid shoulders or recurrent headaches.

Posture is essentially the position of the body in space. Optimal posture is the state of muscular and skeletal balance that protects the supporting structures of the body against injury or progressive deformity, whether at work or rest.

Correct posture involves the positioning of the joints to provide minimum stress on the joints of the body. Conversely, faulty posture increases stress on the joints. Strong muscles can compensate for this increased stress, but if they are weak or the joints lack mobility or are too mobile joint wear and modification can occur. As a result damage and changes to the surrounding tissues can also occur.

Posture also involves the chain-link concept of body mechanics in which problems anywhere along the body chain can lead to problems above or below that point. For example, knee pain can arise from pelvic joint disorders. The effects of posture can be far reaching, involving respiratory, digestive, and circulatory systems as well as the musculoskeletal system.

Improve Your Posture

When you're out at a party, club or even in the office cafeteria, whom do you think people notice first - the guy who is standing tall and straight, or the guy who looks like he wants to crawl into his shell? Well, people may notice the guy who's slouching and looks all curved, but for all the wrong reasons.

It's amazing how something as simple as a good posture can make someone look tall, slim, and most importantly- confident. And the confident man is the one who gets noticed for all the right reasons. So learn how to get your spine all out of a crouch and stand up straight for goodness sake.

Learning how to improve your posture basically consists of knowing how to do it, and having the willpower to stick to it. When we were young, we were told to walk with a book on top of our heads to practice good posture. But now posture starts with three activities we do every day: sitting, standing and sleeping.

Stand up Straight

Look at a mirror while standing up straight. Check out which areas are preventing you from standing up straight: are your shoulders crouched; your head down; your back bent? Straighten out whatever is slouching and observe the difference.

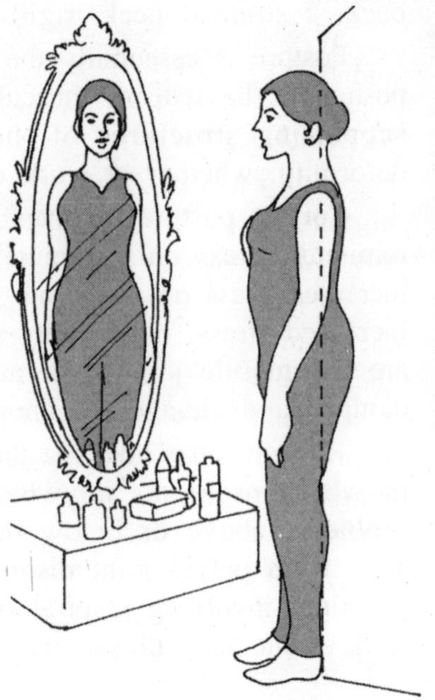

Stand up straight

Your ears, shoulders, hips, knees, and ankles should make one straight line. Relax your shoulders and slightly bend your knees—you don't want to look like a robot.

- Hold the head erect but balanced without tension.
- Hold the chest up and slightly forward, but free to breathe.
- Hold the shoulders well back, but not hunched or strained backward.
- Let the arms hang naturally by the sides.
- Hold the abdomen somewhat flat, or at least not allow it to sag forward. The back will take care of itself if this is done.
- Hold the knees balanced, neither overstretched nor bent.
- Place the feet naturally, with the body weight slightly over the balls of the feet and on the outside edges of the feet. The inside arches of the feet should be held up.

As a posture test, stand facing a wall and 'stretch tall'. Allow your toes to touch the baseboard of the wall. Then lean forward, with your chest jut touching the wall.

You should be able to place both hands, one over the other, between your abdomen and the wall. Now turn around, put your heels to the baseboard and allow your head, shoulders and buttocks to touch the wall.

If you can put your fist between the lower back and the wall, your posture needs improvement.

If you're standing for a long period of time, make sure to continue shifting your weight every so often.

If you're bending down to pick up something, bend your knees and hips, don't bend down and grab the object with just your waist.

Sit Back Regally

Use a high, firm chair with a high back. Make sure to sit with your hips as far back against the back of the chair as possible, and keep your knees at hip level (or a little lower).

If your back is not getting the support it needs from the back of the chair, or you find it difficult to stay against the back of the chair, then try placing a pillow or a towel to support your lower back.

Check how high your shoulders are sitting and how stiff how your neck feels. Many people don't notice that, as they sit still for long periods and their bodies become increasingly rigid and tense, their shoulders become surprisingly raised.

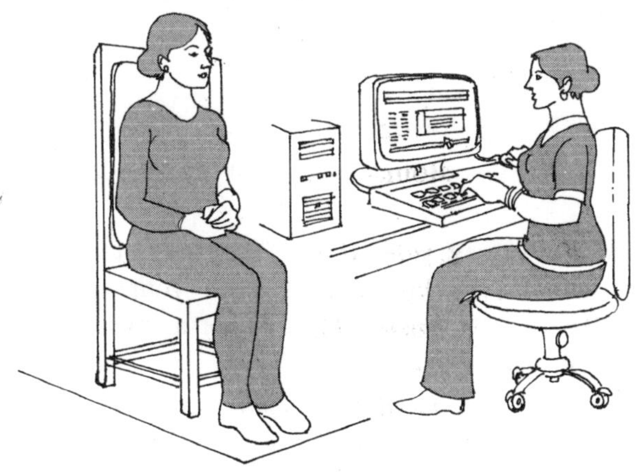

Sit back regally

This seated posture represents the opposite problem to the slouching position, both positions, however, place enormous stress on the back and neck. If you find your body adopting the rigid, tense posture while you're seated, take a couple of deep breaths, and relax your muscles as you exhale. Gently rotate your neck, looking from side to side, and roll your shoulders a couple of times to relax your muscles.

More Tips

- If you're at your desk (working at the computer) all day long, make sure that your workstation is at the height of your elbows.
- Keep your shoulders straight (parallel to your hips) and avoid leaning forward. Remember your entire back should be supported at all times.
- If you find that you're always leaning forward to see your computer monitor, then tilt the monitor upwards so that you're not forced to look down.
- Also, if you usually wear glasses, then try wearing them rather than slouching with your eyes glued to the monitor.
- When driving, make sure to sit straight, with your hips as far back against the back of your chair as possible. You should be able to hold the steering wheel with your elbows slightly bent.
- Avoid staying seated for extended periods of time. Get up and walk around every so often.

Sleep Right, Sleep Tight

Always sleep on a firm mattress.

Don't sleep on your stomach. If you do, place a pillow under your waist.

Sleep on your back or side. If on your back, then you can place a small pillow under your knees; and if on your side, then place a small pillow between your knees. This is not a must, but it may help you maintain a straight back.

Use a pillow for your head that keeps your head aligned (at the same level) with the rest of your body.

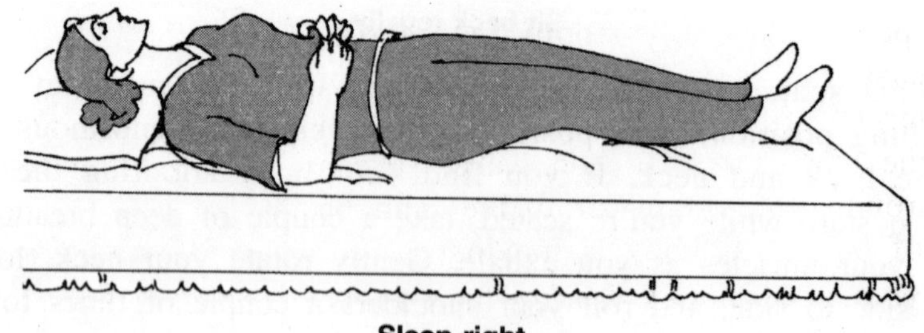

Sleep right

Lift and Carry Without Strain

The size, shape and structure of the material will largely determine how easy or difficult manual handling will be. Whenever you lift a load, make sure that you observe the following rules:

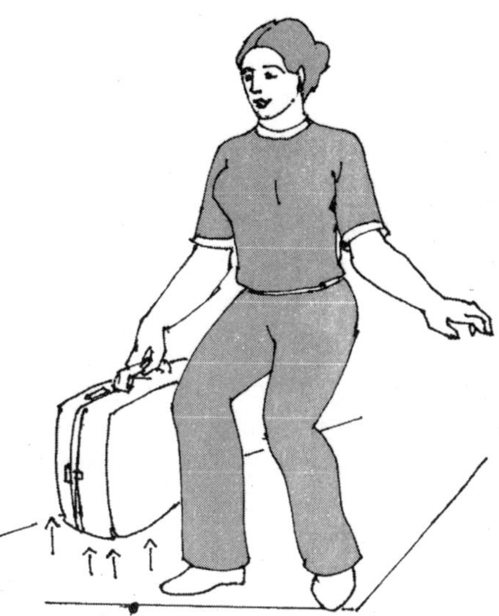

Lift and carry without strain

- Stand close to the load on a firm footing and with feet about 30 cms apart.
- Bend your knees and keep your back as straight as you can.
- Take a firm grip of the load.
- Breathe in and throw the shoulders backward.
- Straighten the legs continuing to keep the back as straight as you can.
- Make sure the load does not obstruct your view.
- Keep the load close to your body.
- Lift slowly and smoothly.
- Once loaded avoid twisting the spine to turn, just move your feet.

Walk Tall

A tall person generally stoops in order to compensate for your height. Regardless of your height, though, think for a moment about the way you stand and walk. Take a walk around your home or office, and be aware of how your body is moving.

If you're a woman wearing high heels, slip them off, and walk barefoot. High heels are, of course, one of the worst offenders

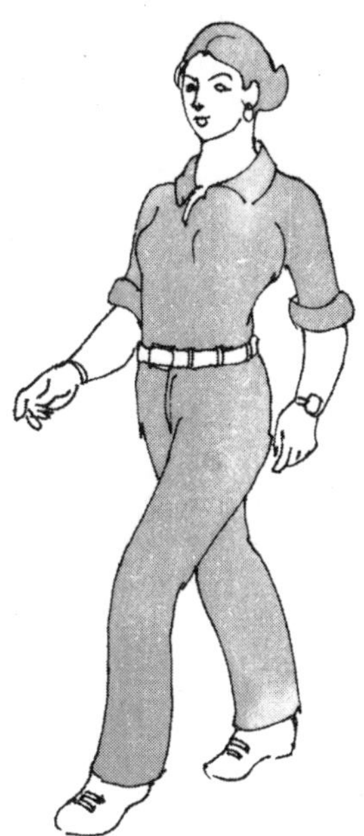

Walk Tall

when it comes to throwing your posture out of line. High shoes tend to pitch the top half of your body forward, as it naturally realigns itself to keep its balance.

As you walk around, try lifting your head until you're looking straight ahead of you, with a relaxed neck and shoulders. Press your shoulders backwards so that your chest is pushed out, and straighten your spine so that you are standing straight, but not too stiffly. You'll notice as you try out this new walk in the privacy of your home or office that you suddenly feel more energetic and confident.

Once you see the difference between slouching along, and striding out, looking directly and confidently at the world, you will want to make a permanent change in the posture you adopt when standing and walking.

Bending

Never bend from the waist, because that will strain your back. Instead, hinge yourself from your true hip joint, which is where your leg meets your torso. Lengthen yourself, floating your head gently up, and hinge from the bottom of your rear.

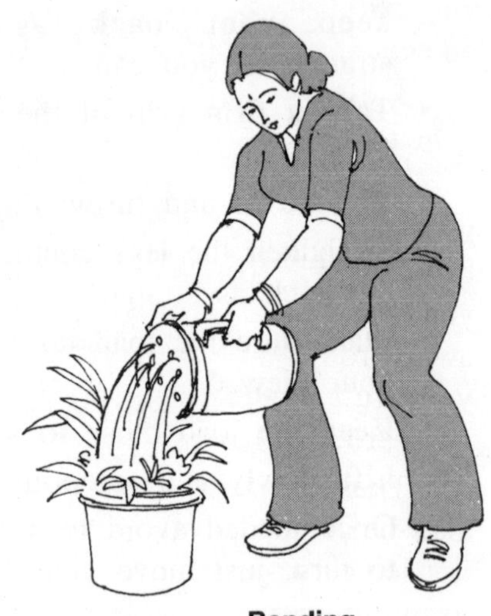

Bending

Squatting

A fine position, as long as you're not hunching over. If you must reach for something, move onto all fours so your reach is well supported. If you tire, you can also sit on the ground, legs spread apart, and work a while that way.

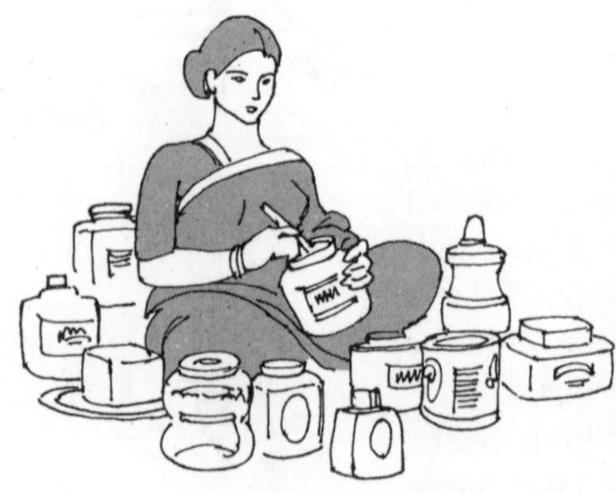

Squatting

Digging

Don't "hunch" when you shovel. Stand up straight, standing over the support of your legs; don't get ahead of yourself. When you move to the side, take a step in the direction you are moving rather than twisting your body.

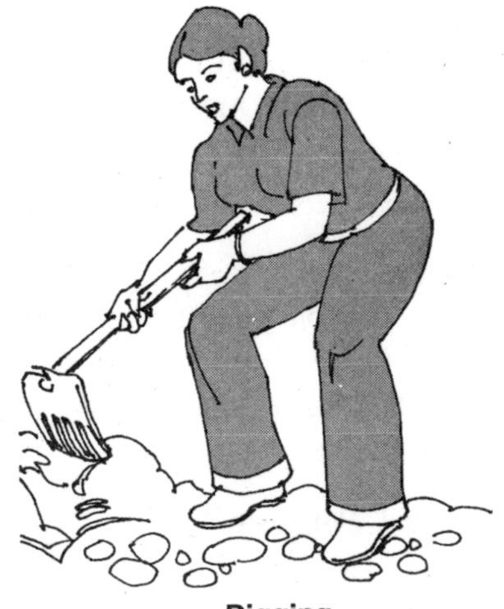

Digging

Lifting

The farther you reach, the wider your stance should be. Get your feet close to the object and use your whole body to lift, rather than just your neck and shoulders, keeping the lifted object close to your body.

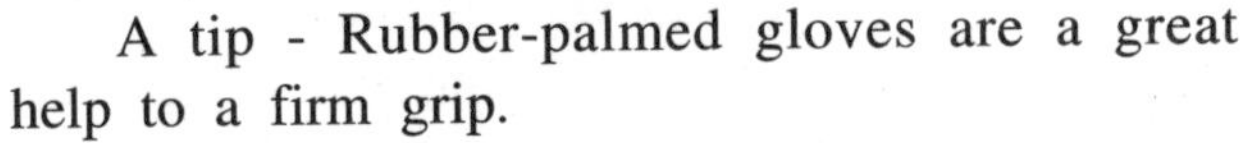

A tip - Rubber-palmed gloves are a great help to a firm grip.

Take frequent breaks, walking away from your task every 10 to 15 minutes, or when you begin to tire. Digging in the dirt can really pull you down, even with the best of intentions. Walk away from your task, coming all the way up to your full dignity, so your whole body moves skyward.

These recommended garden postures could also be applied to a variety of work around the house, especially such activities as scrubbing, vacuuming and dusting.

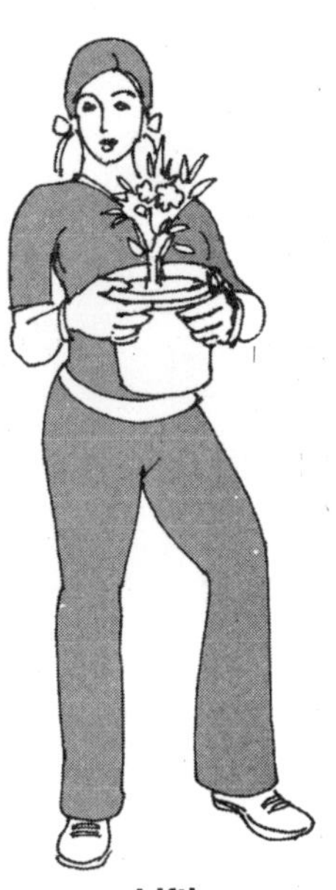

Lifting

Spinal Mobility

The spine is an ingenious feat of engineering capable of movements in all directions: flexion, extension, lateral flexion, and rotation. Combinations of these movements are used on a regular daily basis in common activities. Unfortunately, our sedentary lifestyle has led to dysfunctional posture, which limits the degree of movements possible at the spine.

It is, therefore, important not only to strengthen the muscles of the torso, enabling them to better support the body, but also to improve spinal mobility. Controlled movement through these positions is generally healthy, as it will help maintain full range mobility of the spine.

Spine Stretching

Lying flat on your back, with a book under your head helps lengthen your spine. From this position, slowly bend each leg toward your chest and back again. Then, bring your knees up together and slowly rotate them side-to-side.

Posture Pointers

But the major part of maintaining proper posture is reminding yourself to stand and sit straight. And this is the hardest part. Use these little tips to make sure you don't cheat:

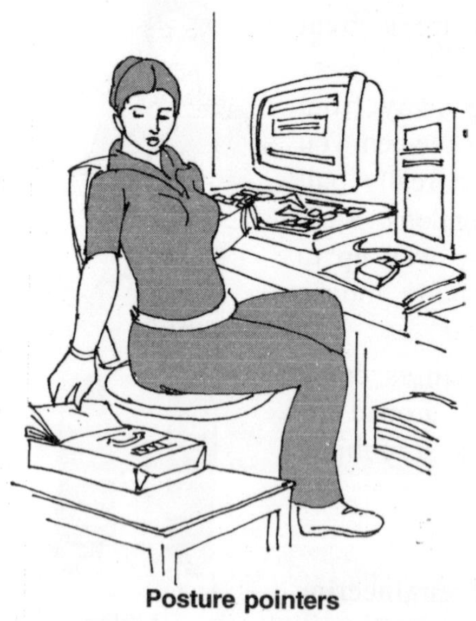

Posture pointers

Tell your friends – They can serve as your support system and they will be glad to elbow you when you're caught slouching. Regular ticking off is bound to stop you from shuffling and slouching.

Use Post-it notes – Put them in areas you see daily; your medicine cabinet mirror, your rear-view mirror, and your computer monitor.

Feel the results – Keep looking at the difference between a good posture and the one you see in the mirror, to really visualize the work to be done.

Exercising often, especially your back and abs, and staying disciplined will reap great physical rewards.

With good posture, you'll be looking thinner, more confident—and you'll have all the reasons in the world to stand tall and be proud.

The Alexander Technique and Posture

Round about the turn of the century, a young Australian actor called Frederick Alexander lost his voice, but only when he was on stage doing his one-man Shakespeare recitals. Doctors couldn't find anything the matter and conventional therapies didn't help. Alexander realised he must be doing something wrong, so he rigged up three mirrors to study himself rehearsing. He saw that when he lifted his head heroically as he recited, he tipped it back, constricting his larynx and incidentally crushing his spinal discs. Yet he could have sworn he'd just been holding his head high.

Once he realised how out of touch people are with what they're actually doing with their bodies, Alexander spent the rest of his life working on his technique.

What Exactly did Alexander Discover?

Basically, he discovered that all of us, when making efforts to do even the simplest things, physical or mental, impose on ourselves harmful tensions that restrict our performance. We are all in the habit of interfering with the natural relationship of the head and neck to the trunk. Observe your own reactions in a tense situation – when driving, perhaps, or during a harassing time at work. Tight muscles pull the head down and clench the jaw, the chest is clamped, restricting breathing, and as the upper body is compressed, the digestive organs or lower back eventually complain. What we popularly call 'bad posture' is often the accumulated residue of all those over-tense reactions that have become locked into the body.

Animals and young children usually move naturally, with a lengthened spine and a sense of poise. Unfortunately, we often acquire bad habits as we get older, and additional stresses can lead to imbalanced and excessive muscular effort in movement. If chronic tensions build up, the neck and back muscles contract, leading to rounded shoulders, a lowered head and an arched back, which causes further tension and so the problem gets worse and worse.

Alexander technique enables you to become more aware of balance, posture and movement in your daily activities and can make you consciously aware of harmful tensions that previously went unnoticed. This involves something that no other therapy offers – learning to stop making unnecessary effort in all kinds of situations.

Alexander students find that the technique not only improves their physical health but also has a considerable impact on personality and outlook, enhancing mental and emotional well-being.

The technique can be helpful in particular for gynaecological conditions, digestive disorders, heart and circulation problems, breathing difficulties, neurological and rheumatic disorders, and psycho-neuroses.

Learning the Technique

In a series of Alexander lessons, the teacher works with a trainee individually, on a one-to-one basis, using his or her hands gently to feel out hidden tensions and distorted muscle pulls and then encouraging the muscles into better balance and harmony. Simple, everyday movement are used as tools for teaching you to move with less tension.

Self-help measures may be of benefit in the first instance; copying Alexander's example and looking closely at your posture in the mirror might be valuable in identifying obvious imbalances. The basic principle of Alexander's ideal posture is to keep your body in a straight line.

The Alexander technique is a way of learning to help yourself, which is one of its great attractions. But it is not a do-it–yourself system–at least not until you have completed a course of lessons. This is because we become accustomed to our own muscle pulls and tensions, and what is familiar comes to feel right even natural. Initially, we must rely on a trained teacher's objective feedback. The teacher will focus on your habits of movement to assess how much strain you impose on yourself. Sitting, rising, standing and lying down are important parts of the lessons. Some of the common features of this technique are listed below:

The Power of Posture

Any distortion to the structure of the spine will affect the way the body works. A hunched posture will inhibit the natural movement of the head, the shoulders and the ribcage, distort the spine and restrict normal breathing patterns. This sagging stance is associated with constantly anxious and depressed people, and it aggravates their feelings of tension. Correct posture is a major step towards improving 'the use of the self'.

Poised and Free

If you examine the way that you sit, either in a large mirror, or with the aid of a teacher, you may see that your habitual positions have already pulled the body down, compressing it, distorting the relation of the head and neck to the trunk. The practised Alexander student will be sitting 'poised and free'. The knees are not crossed since this would twist pelvis and spine.

Rising and Sitting

When you rise from a sitting position your body follows an automatic procedure. Frequently, the head juts forward and the body folds in the middle before straightening upward. The natural curves of the spine are exaggerated. Similarly when sitting down the head is often thrown backward, and the lower back is arched. The Alexander student has a simple and easy rising habit.

Forward and Up

Using a full-length mirror observe yourself standing. The common tendency is to bend the head forward, shortening the neck and rounding the back. The practised student is upright from head to toe; the head is 'forward and up'.

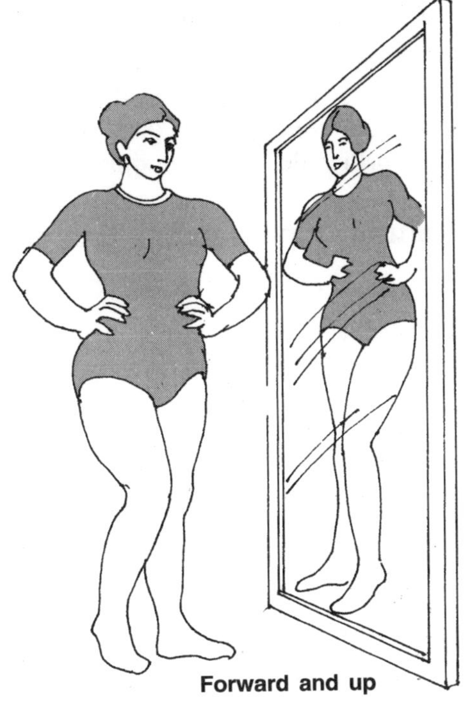

Forward and up

The Alexander technique is a way of becoming more aware of your balance and how you move. It's based on the premise that most people have bad postural habits that, over time, stop us using our bodies as easily and comfortably as we should. Wrongly used muscles contract and pull down, giving in to the classic sign of bad use: head tipped back at the start of any movement, especially sitting or standing. As well as the long-term damage to joints and cramped internal organs, poor posture is linked with respiratory ailments; people develop round shoulders from hunching protectively around their painful chests as they cough and wheeze.

Frederick Alexander believed modern living leads to bad postural habits; shoulders raised and stiffened by stress, neck poked forward over deskwork, tired bodies slumped into saggy armchairs. Soon we've lost all sense of how we really are, so that what feels natural (because it's habitual) is widely out of line. That's why it's hard to correct our own posture without expert help.

The Alexander Technique aims to re-educate the body into moving more easily - relearning the natural grace all children have until they all go to school and start slouching over desks. It's based on what Alexander teachers call 'good use of the body' - allowing the spine to regain its natural curves, holding the head effortlessly in the easiest position and distributing weight evenly over your feet. The bonus is that you look taller and feel lighter.

Most obvious benefits are with back or joint pain, fatigue and respiratory problems. It's also widely used by actors, musicians and athletes to improve their performance. Since there are no risks involved, it's worthwhile trying it out.

Posture Improvement Exercises

Stretching Out

Whether you experience such posture problems at home or at work, some simple stretching exercises can really make a difference to the way your body feels, and remind you to take the time to relax. Try some of these.

Stretch 1

Take off your shoes if you are wearing high heels, and stand with your feet flat on the floor, about shoulder width apart.

Extend both arms to your left and stretch your body gently but fully in that direction. Relax. Repeat the exercise, this time reaching to the right.

Now reach with both hands up towards the ceiling, continuing to look straight ahead. Really reach as hard and as high as you can, extending the stretch until you are standing up on your toes.

Stretch 2

This one is very good for relaxing sore neck and shoulder muscles that have been strained by poor posture.

First move your head slowly to the left, and hold it for a couple of seconds.

Roll your head forward, looking down at your chest, until you are looking towards the right. Be careful not to make any sudden, jerky moves, which will strain your neck muscles further.

Repeat this gentle rolling and stretching motion a few more times, until your neck muscles feel more relaxed.

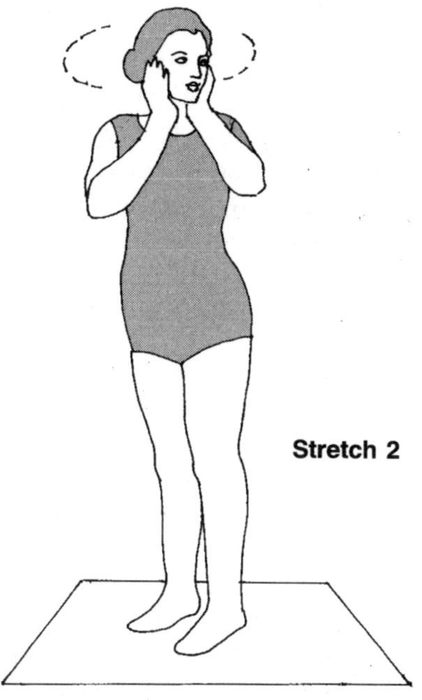

Stretch 2

Shoulder Rolls

Shoulder rolls are also effective remedies for muscles strained by incorrect posture. Make gentle "windmills" with your arms, in a backward direction, five or six times.

Repeat the rolls, this time rotating your arms forward.

Finish off by inhaling deeply, and shrugging your shoulders as high as you can, slowly and thoroughly.

Relax, dropping your shoulders back to their natural level, and exhale fully.

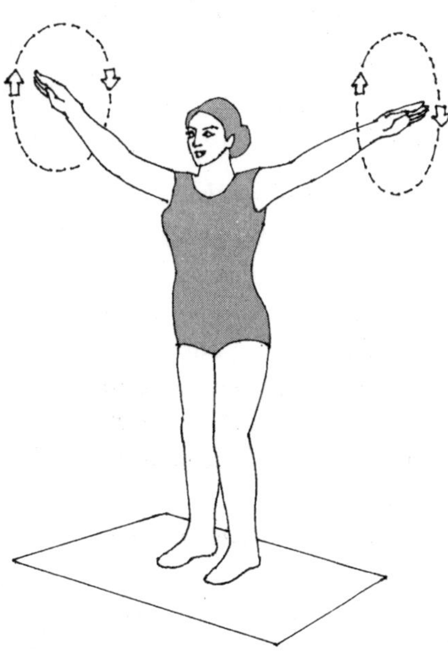

Shoulder rolls

Flexion & Extension

Place your forearms on the floor by your shoulders, push with your forearms and raise your shoulders passively off the ground, as high as is comfortable. It is essential that your shoulders, back and buttocks remain completely relaxed while your arms do all the work. Lower torso to starting position.

Repeat 5-10 times. During back extension, the shoulder blades should be pulled down and together, keeping the shoulders away from the ears. The shoulders should be 'square', not rounded forward.

The prone extension exercise, if properly cued, not only promotes improved range of motion in spinal extension but also helps re-align and establish balance around the shoulder and shoulder girdle.

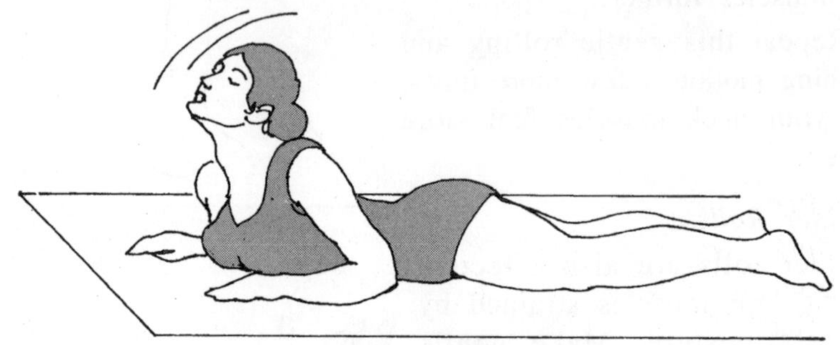

Flexion and extension

Timid Cat Stretch

Kneeling, sitting back on your heels and leaning forwards onto your forearms tuck your head towards your knees and then raise your head high letting your shoulders drop.

Repeat 3-6 times, slowly.

This mobilises the thoracic spine.

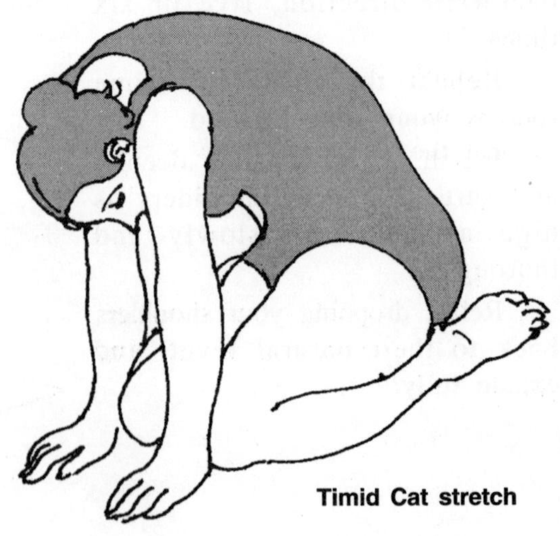

Timid Cat stretch

Single Knee Roll

Lie with one knee bent keeping the foot on the floor and the other leg straight.

Roll the bent knee over the straight leg, pressing it towards the floor and then bring it up again.

Repeat 4-6 times.

Repeat with the other knee.

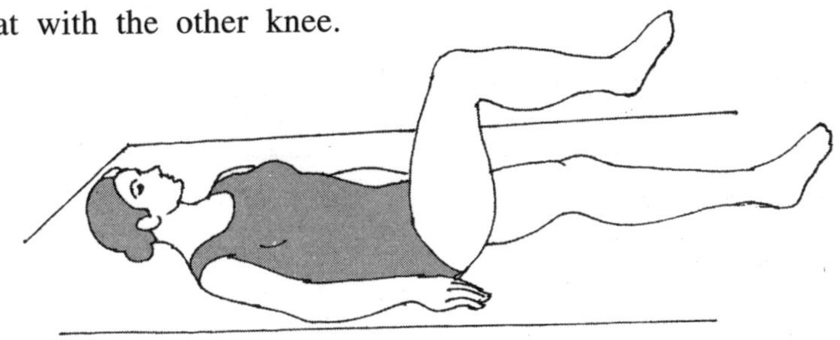

Single knee roll

Side Bend

Standing with your feet together, 10-15 cm from a wall, lean back and rest your back flat against the wall.

Bend to the left stretching your arm down one leg as far as it will go, keeping your entire back and head against the wall.

Gently straighten up.

Repeat 3 times to the left, and then repeat the sequence to the right 3 times.

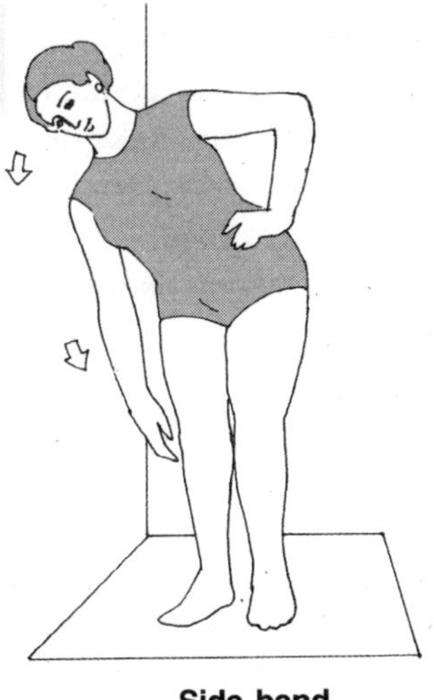

Side bend

■ ■

Chapter 4

YOUTHFUL LOOKS

Everyone wants to look young. Show me a man or a woman who doesn't want to look younger than his or her age and I will show you a liar or a saint.

There was a time when only women bothered about their looks and skin but with changing time it is common to find men going to parlours for a facial treatment and taking as much care of their skin as their female counterpart. It is a good thing, too. Caring about the skin does not make a man less manly, in fact the smooth skin can only add to his charm and personality.

Looking good gives confidence and a sense of enhanced self-esteem, which is essential in today's world. In a world so full of consumerist attitude, good looks are a part and parcel of a personality and to get somewhere one has to be able to make the right impression.

Youthful looks are a result of a healthy lifestyle, which involve a careful regimen of controlled diet, regular exercise and positive thinking. Our face is the mirror of our body and mind. It reflects the healthy conditions we subject our physical and mental as well as emotional faculties to.

Why is it that there are people who have healthy and glowing faces which makes them so beautiful and attractive? On the other hand there are people who age before time, their faces reflecting an unhealthy pallor and a lifetime's exposure to toxic elements. By toxic elements I do not mean the environmental kind only. Toxic elements could be mental as well as emotional ones, too.

The physical grooming of the face and body is just half the battle. To win the entire battle is a monumental job. It requires control over the mind and emotions, too. I will deal with the physical aspect in this chapter; and the mental- emotional well-being will be dealt with in the subsequent chapters.

Supple Skin

Skin is the most important organ in the human body. It regulates the body temperature and performs protective function. Our skin covers the entire body and measures approximately two square yards. Most people do not look beyond the cosmetic aspect in caring for the skin. If one were to observe the skin closely, one would be surprised at the condition of the skin wrought by years of neglect. The ageing process of our skin begins very early in life. The smooth, soft skin of a baby gives way to stressed skin as a result of the daily wear and tear, pollution, age and the regular use of chemically prepared cosmetics on it.

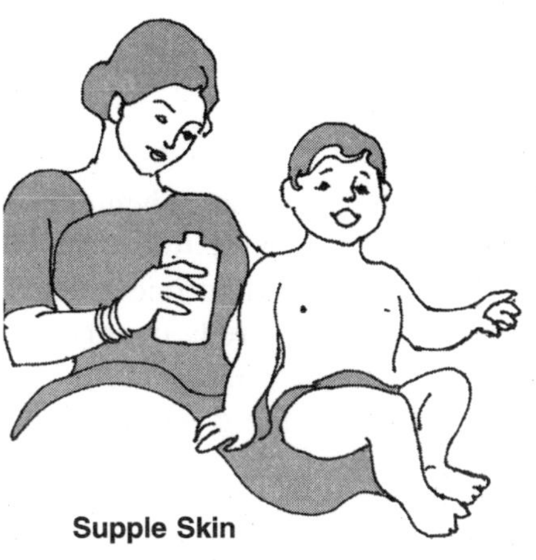

Supple Skin

Skin Phases

Skin is delicate, skin is the mirror of health and skin is what matters... You must have heard it often enough. But did you know that the skin goes through as much upheaval as any other organ, during your lifetime? And that skin requirements and care should change with the years that one has walked on the earth?

Phase I

Teens are the time when the sebaceous glands and oil glands are at their hyperactive peak. The hyperactivity of these glands results in problems like acne, white heads, blackheads, enlarged pores, etc. It is best to live with a scrubbed clean look, which is fresh and young. Natural youthful looks complement the adolescents more than any made up or put on face. The essentials during this phase are a well balanced diet, healthy outlook, positive thoughts and the barest of cosmetics.

Phase II

By the time a person is in the early twenties, the pimple problem has vanished and the skin has settled down to a nice and healthy look. In fact, this is bloom time for the skin. The routine skin care of cleansing, toning, moisturising and nourishing, should keep the skin and complexion looking radiant. If you invest a little time and effort at this stage, you will reap rich rewards in the later years.

Phase III

Thirties is the time, when one has to be on guard. The process of drying out begins at this stage. Fine lines start making their presence felt, and by the time one reaches late thirties the skin begins to look rather dull and tired, if adequate care has not gone into the health routine. Premature ageing is a real threat and one can retard the process by keeping away from direct sun.

Phase IV

The skin can really become dull and tired by the time a person reaches the forties. The sebaceous glands slow down and produce less oil, which leads to dryness and wrinkles. The collagen fibres begin to thin, and the skin's ability to hold moisture also reduces. The elasticity and the suppleness of the skin are impaired. Hormonal imbalances in the late forties can play havoc with the health of the skin. Crow's feet and laughter lines deepen, and the furrow between the brows is accentuated. The skin pores enlarge, leading to an uneven texture. It is imperative that measures like facials, packs and proper nourishment, supplement the regular beauty routine. Regular exercises and a balanced diet, along with meditation to calm the mind, can really help at this stage.

Phase V

The fifties need not be dreaded; although it is a visibly tired skin that greets the eyes each time one looks at the mirror. The fat deposits under the skin diminish, lending it a flabby appearance. The skin also gets drier and loses elasticity. There is a leathery look and the complexion becomes mottled. At the same time, it is not rare to find a woman at her glowing best during this stage. This radiance does not come from beauty regimen, alone. It is also the result of being at peace with the realities of life. Apart from regular beauty care, it is important to develop a positive, peaceful attitude, and incorporate a regimen of regular exercise in the lifestyle.

From the teens to late sixties is a long road for the skin. It goes through many upheavals of physical, emotional and environmental kind. A beauty regimen alone cannot help. Good diet, regular exercise, positive attitude and a healthy outlook go a long way in keeping it glowing through the years.

Ageing Factors

Although it is natural for the skin to age with the biological clock, certain factors can accelerate the rate of ageing.

- Smoking
- Drinking alcohol
- Excessive caffeine consumption
- Excessive exposure to sun
- Stressful living
- Deficient diet
- Lack of exercise
- Insomnia
- Environmental pollution

Dry Skin and Wrinkles

We all know that the skin changes with age. It is one of life's universal laments. The most common manifestation of these changes is dryness of the skin. This drying of the skin emphasizes wrinkles, and contributes to flaking, cracking and itching. Although dry skin is a natural consequence of ageing, it can usually be controlled with simple, easy-to-follow measures that help to keep it moist and young looking.

A decrease in the secretions from oil and sweat glands is seen with ageing. These secretions originate in the *dermis* (the innermost layer of skin) and reach the *epidermis* (the outermost layer of skin) through pores that lead to the surface.

Once the secretions emerge, the oil traps sweat (which is primarily composed of water) just under the exposed surface of the epidermis. As a result, the skin retains moisture and remains well hydrated.

Oil and water secretions are abundant during the teen years and early adult life, but over the years these secretions lessen and the skin gradually dries out.

Other factors, which contribute to the problem, include thinning of the skin with ageing, as well as loss of the fat and supporting connective tissue.

Cold weather, dry air, bathing too frequently, using harsh skin care products and allergic reactions can also be the contributing factors.

Keep Your Skin Healthy

Keeping your skin well hydrated will improve its appearance and keep it healthy. The following suggestions are effective, inexpensive and easy to implement.

1. ***Avoid direct sunlight*** – In addition to causing dryness, sun exposure is the leading cause of skin cancer. It is best to minimise sun exposure, especially during the peak hours of 10 a.m. and 3 p.m. when the sun's rays are the most intense. A wide brim hat is a useful tool to block direct sunlight exposure.
2. ***Daily use of sunscreen*** – Routine use of a sunscreen will prevent the damaging effects of the sun as well as minimise the drying effects of the sun. For regular use, a S.P.F. (Sun Protection Factor) of 15 is adequate. A higher S.P.F. of 30 to 45 is recommended for high sun exposure activities such as snow skiing or travel to the beach.
3. ***Bathe only once daily*** – Bathing more frequently can worsen dryness of the skin by stripping away the natural protective oils of the skin. Although bathing more than once a day may seem to relieve itching at first, it is counter-productive in the long run. Hot water should also be avoided in an effort to minimise drying of the skin.
4. ***Cautious use of bath oil*** – Although bath oil is an effective moisturiser, adding it to bath water is dangerous because it makes the tub slippery. Also, the residue may be difficult to clean from

the tub. If you do use bath oil, add it to the water after you've been soaking for 15 minutes, otherwise the oil will coat your body and prevent the water from penetrating the skin. A safer use of bath oils is to smooth it on the skin after you get out of the tub.

5. ***Use mild soaps*** – Only mild soaps with moisturising contents should be used; otherwise it is best to use a face wash.
6. ***Pat yourself dry*** – Vigorous rubbing disrupts the smooth skin surface. Gently patting of the skin is much less irritating and will decrease drying, flaking and cracking of the skin.
7. ***Use a humidifier*** – Low humidity will dry the skin. The lower the humidity, the faster the skin will lose water. If the air in your home is dry, a humidifier can raise humidity and slow dehydration of the skin.
8. ***Using the air conditioner*** – The air conditioner has a drying effect on the skin. The difference in the temperature, when you step out from the air-conditioned interiors to the natural environment, has a devastating effect on the skin.
9. ***Tone up the skin*** – toning is the process of balancing dry and moist patches of skin, neutralizing the chemicals and giving the skin an even tone. In addition, a toner removes all traces of excess oil.
10. ***Moisturise*** – You should moisturise at least once daily. The best time to moisturise is immediately after bathing because that's when the moisturiser can trap the water into the skin. Moist skin is a happy skin, so always moisturise your skin even if it is oily skin. It is a good idea to let your skin breathe while you sleep, so wash your face about half an hour after applying moisturiser so it would have absorbed a sufficient amount of moisture by the time you wash it off.
11. ***See a dermatologist*** – The dermatologist has the final key to a youthful skin. Alpha hydroxy acids as well as Retin-A creams have been shown to reverse the signs of ageing and return a more youthful appearance to the skin. Laser therapy, which can remove liver warts, age spots, spider veins, broken blood vessels, red blotches or birthmarks, can also remove years from your appearance.

Persistent dryness, itching, eczema, blisters or sores should be evaluated by a dermatologist, as this may be an indication of a more serious medical condition such as cancer, liver disease, kidney disease, diabetes, thyroid disease, lupus or anemia.

Facial Exercises

Are you tired of wrinkles and an ageing face? The panacea lies in doing certain exercises for the face. Facial exercises can be effective in keeping you looking young since they prevent the slackening of facial muscles

Benefits of Facial Exercises

Never mind how good your skin care might be, there will be a time in your life when all your facial muscles simply go slack, lax, saggy, baggy and crepey. Facial exercises are economical - they do not take great effort or too much time, and pay handsome dividends in achieving a more smooth, with less wrinkles, lines and bags, resulting in a skin that is glowing with health and vitality.

An ageing face has lines, wrinkles, folds and bags which are nothing but the supportive muscles in your face going soft - losing their firmness, and not supporting the skin any more. Facial exercises can help with this problem by creating the facelift you might need, with a non-surgical procedure.

Facial exercises are not only for mature people to achieve a youthful, young, ageless and anti-ageing face - but also for young people to maintain their youthful looks. They can be started at any age, in fact, sooner the better because they act as a deterrent to the formation of wrinkles and other lines on the face.

Contrary to what some people believe, facial exercises do not cause wrinkles if done correctly - they actually help to make women and men look younger for longer, without a surgical facelift, by toning facial muscles. Surgical facelifts can be effective, but are expensive, and can be traumatic.

Tone up the Facial Muscles

A droopy double chin, or a couple of double chins, hanging cheeks, puckered up mouth, puffy and droopy eyelids - does this sound familiar? If it does, you definitely should get down to work.

The facial muscles are connected to the skin and the bone, and form the "cushion" on which the skin rests. If this cushion is flat, worn-out, compressed and not consistent in thickness, the skin will also not look its best. The facial exercises not only benefit the supportive muscles, but also improve the skin, and tone, as the increased blood flow assists in bringing nutrition to, and removing toxins from the skin.

The elasticity and health of the skin is determined to a large extent on the underlying tone, strength and vitality of the supporting facial muscles. Facial muscle exercises, just like body muscle exercises must be done regularly to achieve and maintain results. To get your facial muscles toned up, do these facial exercises daily, for at least a month, or until the desired effect is achieved, and then do these exercises at least three times a week to maintain the results.

Some people report that minor spots or blemishes appear after starting facial exercises, this effect is normal. Since the skin is once again stimulated to produce its natural oils and lubricants, these minor spots may appear when starting facial exercises, until the skin is functioning efficiently and correctly again. Cells get lazy and stagnate, but with proper exercises these cells are once again activated to work with renewed vigour.

The appearance of your skin relies in part on the supportive muscles and in order for these muscles to be well toned, firm and help project a vibrant and youthful face, they need to be exercised and well toned.

Exercises for the Neck

Here are some facial exercises that you might find useful in your quest for a smooth and ageless face, without any surgical facelift. Like normal exercises, facial exercises need to be done regularly to achieve and get the full benefit from it. A double chin and "untidy" neck and throat can give an ageing look. Some people might think that a double chin is simply excess weight manifesting itself, but what they don't realise is that it also is the manifestation of loose skin and terrible muscle tone.

My mother used to say that in order to ascertain a person's age, look at their neck. There is nothing nice or pretty about a lined neck with loose skin hanging around. These exercises are designed to relieve and prevent a double chin, tighten up the loose skin in the neck and throat area and will also assist in toning these muscles.

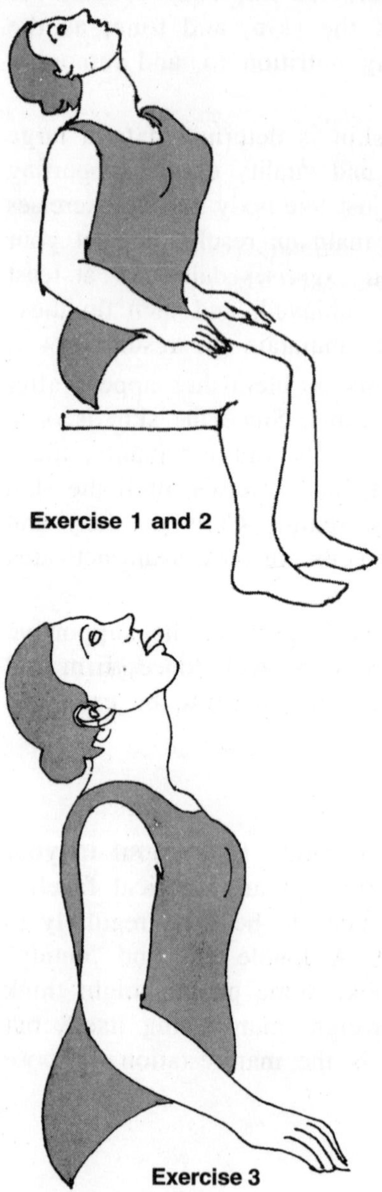
Exercise 1 and 2

Exercise 3

Exercise 1

Sit upright, tilt your head back looking at the ceiling, while keeping your lips closed and then start a chewing movement.

You will feel the muscles working in your neck area. Repeat 20 times.

Exercise 2

Sit upright, tilt your head back looking at the ceiling, while keeping your lips closed and relaxed. Start puckering your lips together in a kiss and stretch the kiss, as if you were trying to kiss the ceiling.

Keep your lips puckered for 10 counts, then relax, bring your head back to normal and repeat 5 times.

Exercise 3

Sit upright, tilt your head back looking at the ceiling, while keeping your lips closed and relaxed. Open your lips and stick your tongue out as if you were trying to touch your chin with the tip of your tongue.

Keep your tongue out in this position for 10 counts, and return your tongue and head to their normal position.

Exercise 4

Sit upright, tilt your head back looking at the ceiling, while keeping your lips closed and relaxed. Next move your lower lip over your top lip as far as possible and keep it there for a count of 5. Relax and repeat 5 times.

Exercise 5

Lie on your bed, with your head hanging down over the edge. Slowly bring your head up towards your torso and keep it there for 10 counts.

Relax and lower your head towards the floor again. Repeat 5 times.

Exercise 6

Sit upright and face forward and while keeping your lips together, separate your teeth by dropping your jaw and then push your jaw forward, keep for a count of 10.

Bring the jaw back to starting position and repeat 5 times.

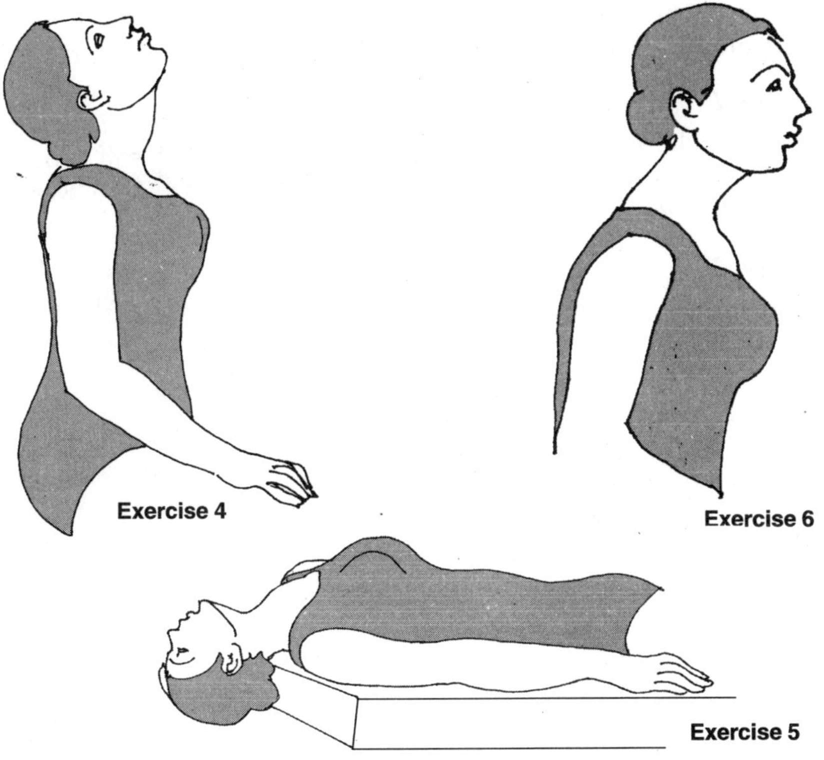

Eye and Forehead Exercises

Eyes are the windows to our souls, and it is better to surround your eyes with firm, smooth unlined skin, than to surround it with wrinkles, lines, character lines, crow's feet or laughter lines. When we talk to people they tend to focus their attention on the eye-area. A tired looking and lined area around the eyes can add years to the face.

These facial exercises deal with baggy eyes, puffy eyes, droopy eyelids, wrinkles on your forehead and eyebrows.

• Eye Exercises

The area around the eye is of the thinnest and most fragile kind found on the body, and wrinkles in this area can give an ageing look to the face. Bags under the eyes also do great disservice to your looks and create an un-cared for look.

Baggy eyes can be helped with certain facial eye exercises, but baggy eyes can also be caused by a multitude of factors, which exercising may not resolve or sort out. Droopy eyelids can, however, benefit greatly from these facial exercises.

Exercise 1

Gently tone the muscles of the eyes by pressing two fingers on each side of your head, at the temples, while opening and closing your eyes rapidly. Repeat 5 times.

Exercise 2

Sit upright with your eyes closed and relaxed. While keeping your eyes closed, first look down and then look up as far as possible.

Repeat this exercise 10 times.

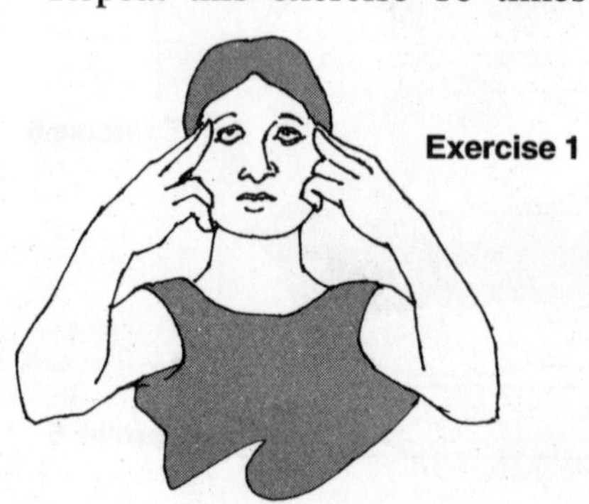

Exercise 1

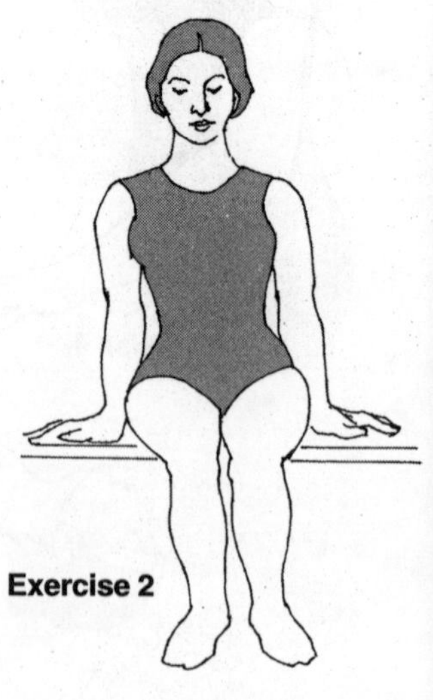

Exercise 2

Exercise 3

Sit upright with your eyes closed and relaxed. Keep your eyes closed while lifting your eyebrows and stretching your eyelids down as far as possible.

Keep in this position for 5 counts, relax and repeat 5 times.

Exercise 4

Sit upright with your eyes relaxed and open. Lift your eyebrows while closing your top eyelids until about halfway closed, then open your eyelid wide open until the white of your eye shows over your iris.

Exercise 5

Sit upright looking straight ahead with your eyes open.

Look up then down, while keeping your head still. Repeat 10 times.

Then look left and right - repeat 10 times.

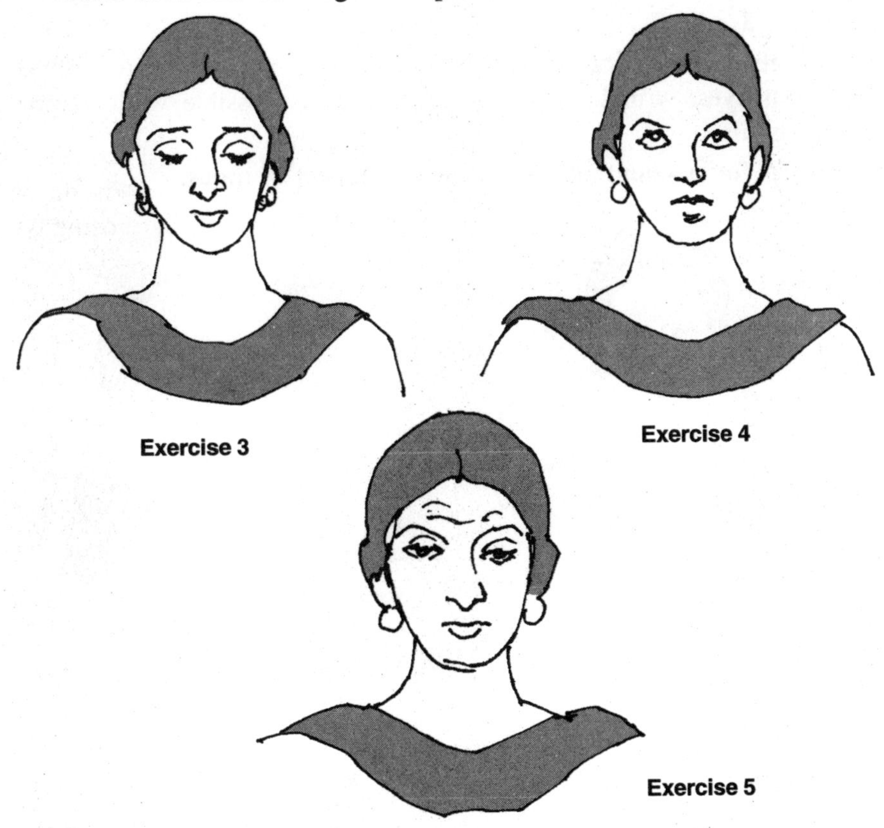

Exercise 3

Exercise 4

Exercise 5

• Forehead Exercises

The area on the forehead, between the eyebrows, can easily become lined and full of wrinkles. These exercises can be a great help in preventing the formation of these wrinkles.

Exercise 1

Frown as much as possible and try to bring your eyebrows over your eyes while pulling the eyebrows towards one another.

Then lift your eyebrow as far as possible while opening your eyes as wide as possible. Repeat 5 times.

Exercise 2

Lie on your bed with your head hanging over the edge. Lift your eyebrows as high as possible, with your eyes open very wide. Relax and repeat 10 times.

Exercise 3

Sit upright facing forward and while bringing your eyebrows down over your eyes, wrinkle your nose as far up as possible while flaring your nostrils.

Keep for a count of 10, relax and repeat 5 times.

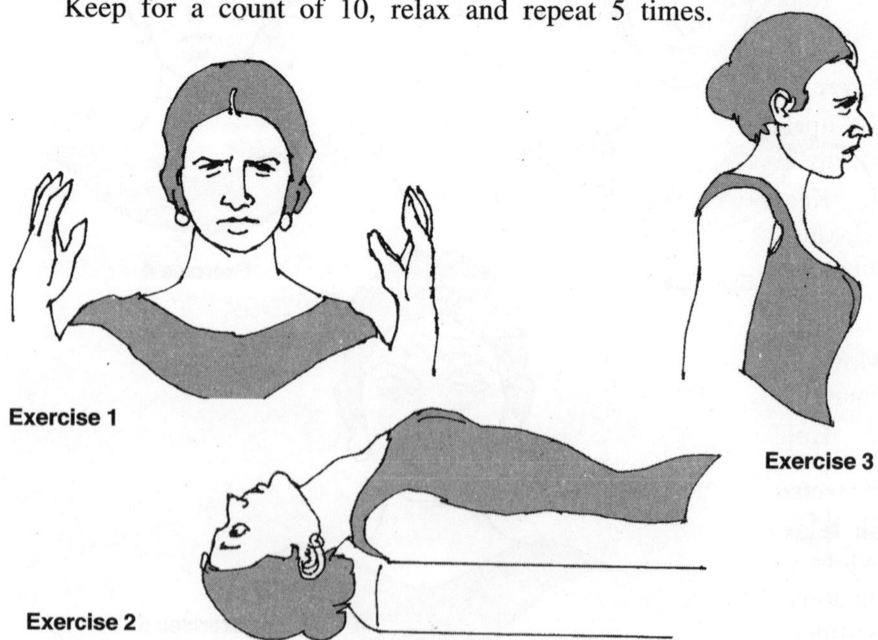

Lips and Cheeks Exercises

If the skin around your mouth is puckered and lined, it not only gives you a bitter look, but also adds years to your visual age. A "bitter" mouth with grim lines and furrows are the "look" of a positive and vital person, and sagging jowls and cheeks might look good on certain dogs, but definitely not on humans.

These exercises are effective in dealing with wrinkled and lined lips as well as lined and sagging cheeks.

- **Exercises for the Lips**

Exercise 1

Sit upright facing forward and purse your lips together. Lift your pursed lips towards your nose and keep them there for 5 counts, relax and repeat 5 times.

Exercise 2

Pucker your lips slightly and in this puckered position try with your mouth muscles to bring the corners of your mouth together as close as possible.

Keep the lips in this position for 5 counts, relax and repeat 5 times.

Exercise 3

Sit upright, facing forwards and keep your lips closed and teeth together. Smile as broadly as possible, without opening your lips.

Keep it in that position for 5 counts. When the muscles begin relaxing pucker your lips in a pointed kiss. Hold for 5 counts and relax. Repeat 10 times.

Exercise 4

Move your lips into a puckered kiss and while relaxing the kiss keep your lips closed and curl your lips into your mouth across your teeth.

Hold this position for a count of 10 and repeat 5 times.

Exercise 5

Sit relaxed with your lips barely open and pucker your lips outwards. While your lips are in the outward position, move your puckered top lip towards your nose. Hold in this position for 10 counts and repeat 5 times.

Exercises for the Lips

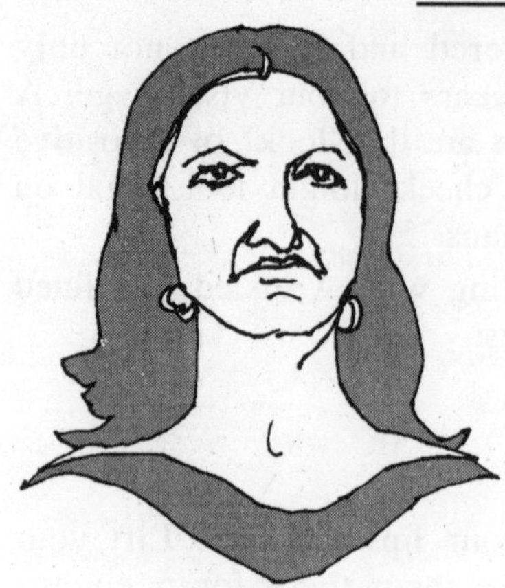

Exercise 1

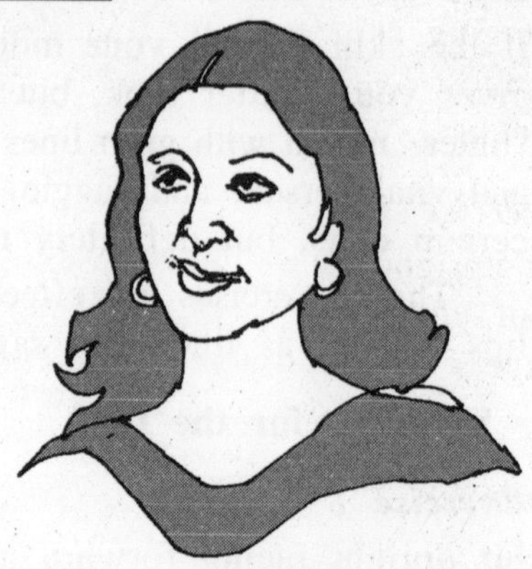

Exercise 2

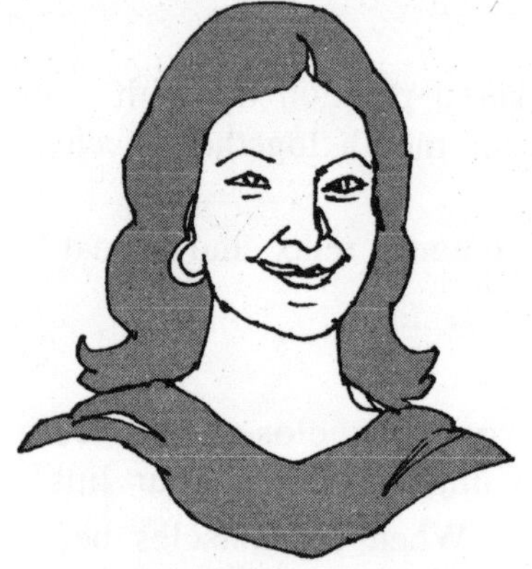

Exercise 3

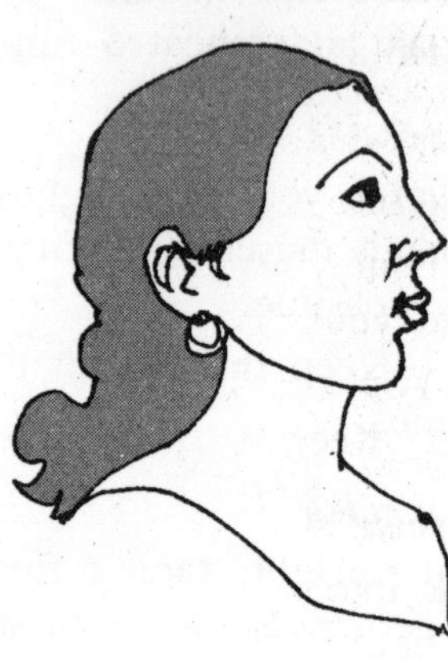

Exercise 4

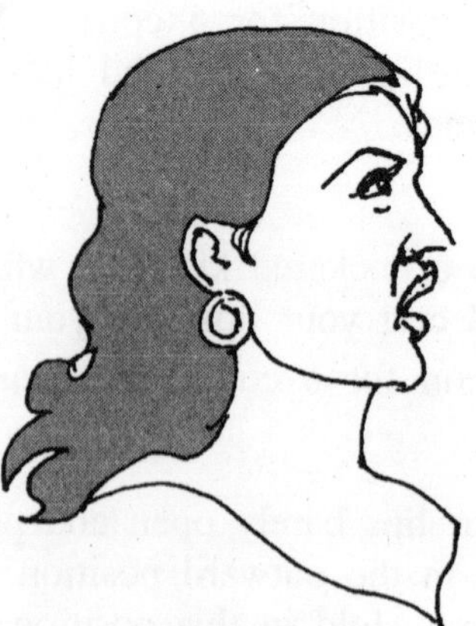

Exercise 5

• **Exercises for the Cheeks**

Hanging skin forming that hang-dog look around your cheeks can be most ageing. Here are some facial exercises to lift and firm the cheeks.

Exercise 1

Sit upright facing forward with lips closed but relaxed. Pucker and pout your lips using the muscles in your cheeks. (Feel with your fingers for the tightening of the cheek muscles)

Keep it puckered for a count of 10, relax and repeat 10 times.

Exercise 2

Relax your face into a smile with your lips closed and then suck in your cheeks towards and on to your teeth.

Hold this for 10 counts, relax and repeat 10 times.

Exercise 3

Look into a mirror while doing this exercise.

Pout your top lip, turning the corners of your lips upward and move your cheek muscles towards your eyes.

You should at this stage try to get your top lip touching your nose. Keep in this position for 10 counts, relax and repeat 5 times.

Exercise 4

Look into a mirror while doing this exercise.

Smile a wide as possible - while keeping your lips closed and your mouth corners turned up.

Try to make your mouth corners touch your ears. Next wrinkle your nose and see your cheeks muscle move upwards and feel these muscles work.

Hold this position for 5 counts, relax and repeat 10 times.

Exercise 5

Keeping your teeth and lips closed, blow air under your top lip and keep it there for 10 counts, then move it to your left cheek's side.

Hold for 10 counts then blow air under your lower lip.

Hold for 10 counts and then blow air into your right cheek while holding it for a count of 10. Repeat 5 times.

Exercises for the Cheeks

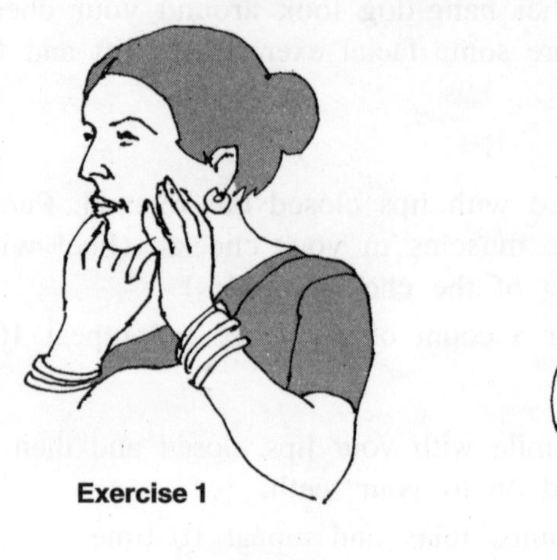

Exercise 1

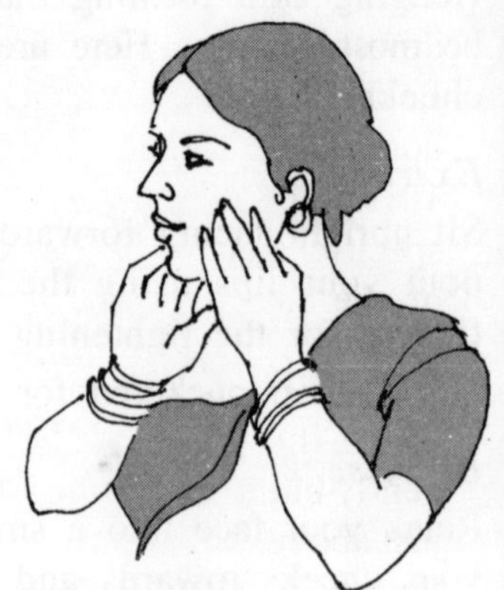

Exercise 2

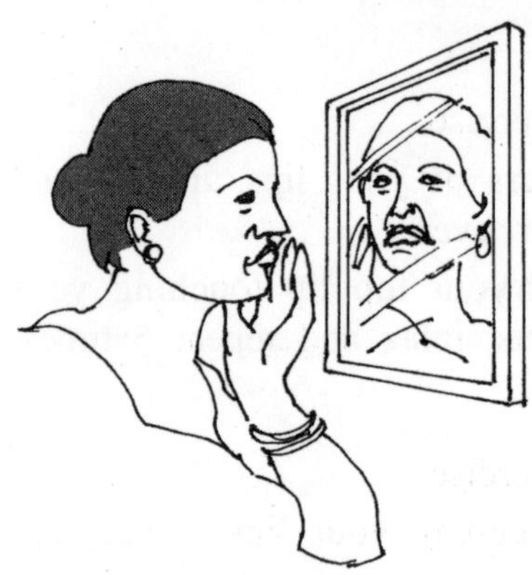

Exercise 3

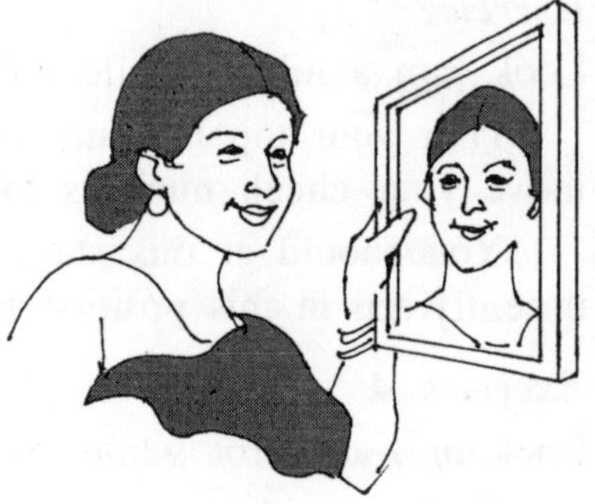

Exercise 4

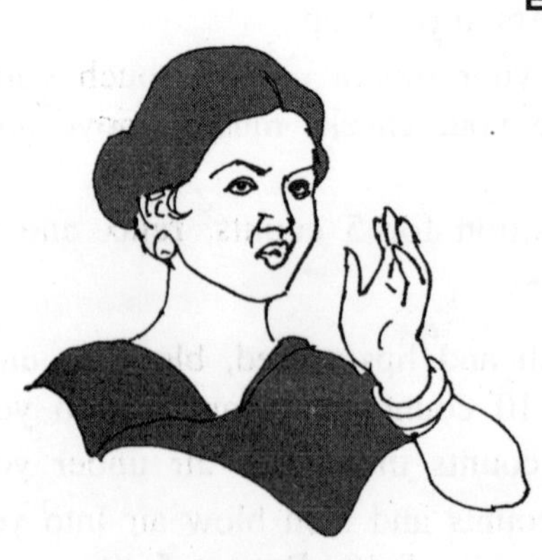

Exercise 5

Some More Facial Exercises

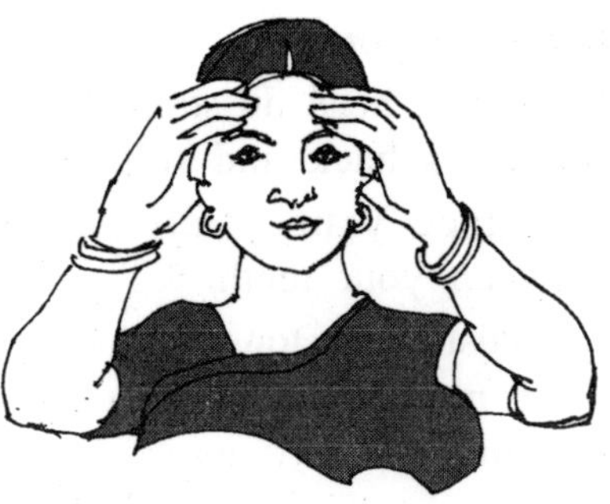

Horizontal forehead lines

These exercises are designed to develop tone for the facial muscles. Each of these exercises should be done for 6 seconds and repeated for 10 minutes a day. Work on the specific area while keeping the rest of the face relaxed.

Horizontal Forehead Lines

Place the sides of the forefingers gently but firmly against the forehead just above the eyebrows, allowing the thumbs to rest lightly on the cheeks.

Raise the eyebrows against the resistance of the fingers.

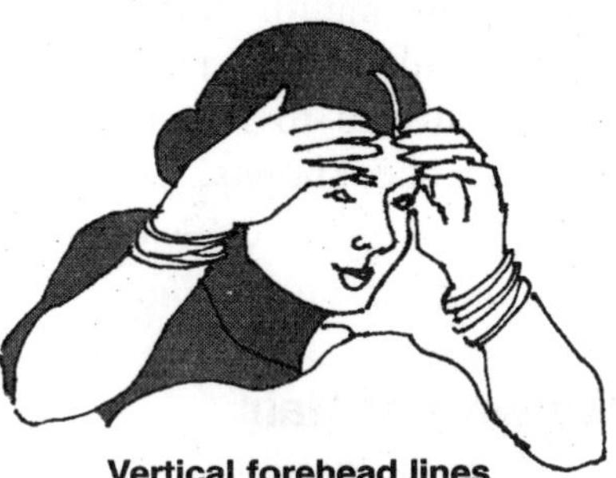

Vertical forehead lines

Vertical Forehead Lines

Place the underside of the forefingers flat against the forehead just above the eyebrows and pull gently towards the temple.

Eyes

Raise your eyebrows, lower your eyes and hold them at half open position for 10 seconds and relax.

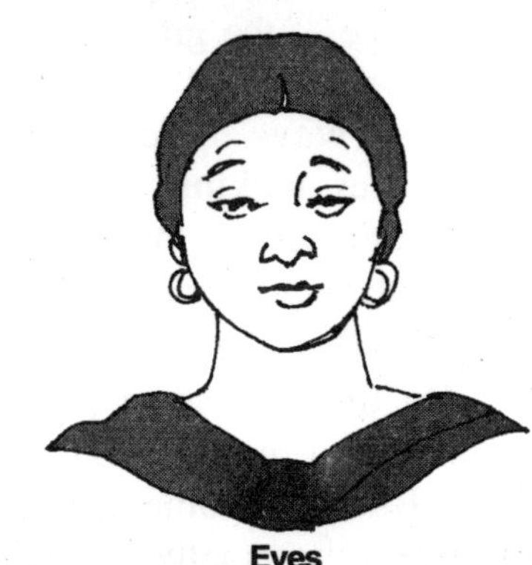

Eyes

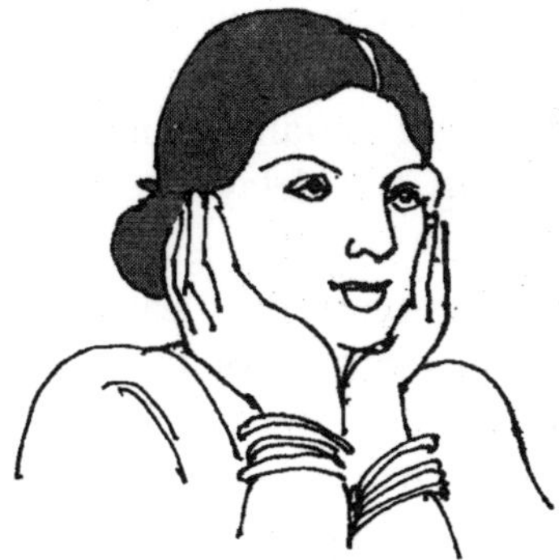

For the laugh lines

For the Laugh Lines

Place the hands flat on the cheeks with the finger-tips touching the cheek-bones and the wrists meeting together.

Gently pull towards the ears. Holding this position say 'You'.

Droopy Chin

Hold your head up straight, chin level and shoulders back and relaxed.

Place your forefinger horizontally between your teeth.

Push your tongue against the roof of your mouth while keeping your teeth touching your finger.

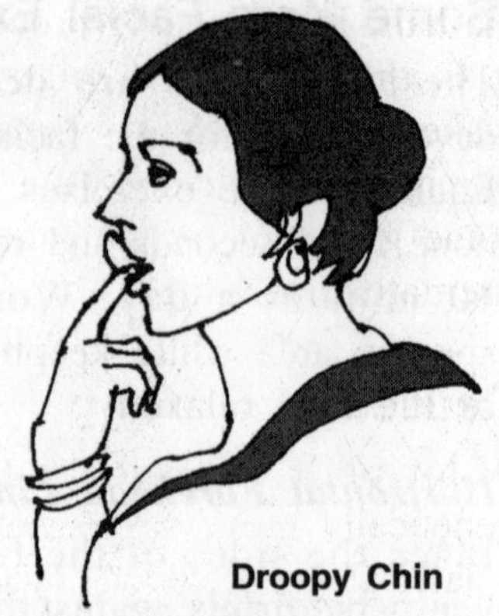

Droopy Chin

Neck

With your mouth half open, place your palms under your jaw and curve your fingers around to rest lightly on the side of your cheekbones.

Try to open your mouth against the resistance of your hands.

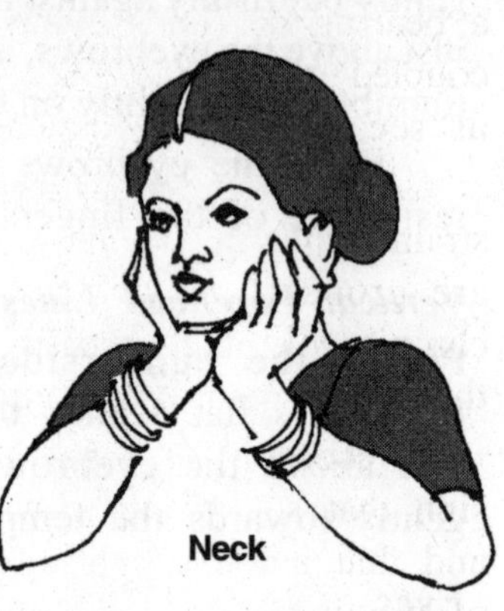

Neck

Greying of Hair

One of the first signs of ageing is the appearance of the grey hair. It is something most people dread and fear. They adopt various ways and means to keep themselves looking young through hair-dyes. Although in the earlier generations the appearance of grey hair was in the age group of forties, today it can be seen in much younger people. Often boys and girls as young as 25 have grey hair.

Up till now, most people accepted greying as an inevitable part of the ageing process. One can either live with it or cover it with hair dyes. But now some experts are suggesting that certain changes in lifestyle can actually prevent premature greying and delay the entire process.

The greying of hair is known as *palitya* in Ayurveda. Each hair has a root, a stem or a shaft and sprouts from the base of the scalp. The stem varies greatly in thickness, from person to person. What is strange is that it is rounded in normal straight hair while curly hair has an oval or flattened section. The different colour of the hair is caused by pigment (pigment) scattered in varying amounts throughout the hair. In the ageing process the hair bulb produces less hair pigment. It is the absence of pigment in the cortical layer of the hair that makes the hair clear (or grey). What exactly is the reason for the lack of pigment formation is a mystery. About 88% people claim to have some grey hair by the time they are 40, of that some 1% suffer from premature greying.

Causes of Greying

A lot of it depends on the genes of a person. Some people are genetically prone to premature greying while others may not grey till a later stage. Regional factors like food habits and weather also have a bearing on the greying of hair. High levels of stress and anxiety coupled with a fast pace of life may also accelerate the process. Let us see what ayurveda has to say about the process of greying.

According to Ayurveda excessive passion, anger and psychic strain results in greying of hair. Persons with *pittika* type of constitution are prone to be affected by this ailment. Persons suffering from chronic cold and sinusitis and those who use warm water for washing their hair are more likely to be victims of this condition.

According to naturopaths, premature greying can be an outward sign that something is wrong with the internal balance of the body, and that a number of lifestyle factors can contribute to the process of greying. These include factors like stress, alcohol consumption, smoking and recreational drugs because these lead to a build up of acidity in the body tissues, which makes it difficult for the body to process the B vitamins efficiently. These vitamins are directly linked to hair colour and are important for the creation of colour pigmentation cells.

High levels of stress can contribute to the premature greying of hair. Sudden shocks can also accelerate the process since people under stress use up more B vitamins.

Ayurvedic Remedies

This is a question most of us would like to have answers to. Apart from using hair dyes, there are hardly any other remedies to the greying syndrome. But there are many medicines prescribed in Ayurveda that are said to arrest premature greying of hair.

Here are a few of them:—

- Take one-teaspoonful of *amrita* (giloya), *amla* and *gokhroo* mixed in equal parts to which honey is added, thrice a day.
- Grind into powder two parts of *bhringaraja,* one part of back sesame seeds, and one part of *amla.* Take a teaspoonful of the powder with milk and sugar. This however has to be continued for some months before the effects are visible.
- For the impatient who want faster results, *swarnamakshika bhasma* may be added in 240 mg doses with the powders.
- Use *bhringaraja taila* (hair oil) regularly. *Eladi taila* can also be used for massaging the scalp.
- Grind into paste equal quantities of old *mandur, amla,* and *jaba* (Hibiscus rosa sinensis) flowers and apply it on the head. After the paste dries, wash hair with water in which amla his been soaked overnight.
- Grind together into fine powder: *amla*-two parts, *harada*-two parts, *bahera*-one part, stone of *mango*-five parts, and old *mandur*-two and half parts. Make a paste of a teaspoonful of this powder with water in which amla has been soaked overnight. Keep this overnight in an iron vessel and apply it to the hair in the morning. After it dries, apply oil to the hair and then wash thoroughly.

The naturopathic solution to the problem lies in creating the right pH or acidity level in the body. This means reducing the intake of meat and animal fats and eating a diet rich in alkaline foods such as carrots, celery, almonds, figs, endive, fruit, green vegetable and wheat-grass.

One also has to make changes in the lifestyle, which include giving up smoking, improving the diet etc. You can slow the greying process, and even restore the hair to its natural colour through these changes, claim naturopaths.

Anti-Greying Diet

Diet has a very important role in preventing and arresting premature greying of hair.

Eating a lot of fruits and vegetables is absolutely essential to facilitate the supply of essential vitamins and minerals. Since the link between lack of B vitamins and greying has been established almost definitely, it is necessary to consume foods that provide these vitamins.

Foods like wheat germ and pulses, whole grains, brewer's yeast, nuts, fortified breakfast cereals, liver, milk, kidney, dairy products, wheat bran, wheat germ, eggs, peanuts, legumes, meat and fish, dark green leafy vegetables, avocados, walnuts, pork, poultry, bananas, and potatoes which belong to the B vitamin group, should be taken in plenty to retard the greying process.

Where it is not possible to consume a diet rich in these vitamins, a supplement containing B vitamins can be taken daily, in order to compensate the shortfall. But one has to keep in mind that the supplement should contain all the vitamins in the B group.

Anti-Ageing Wonder Called Vitamin E

In the recent years, science has discovered a wonder called Vitamin E which can effectively slow down the ageing process by keeping the skin healthy and glowing, the hair glossy, and provide a boost to the immunity system.

A process called oxidation, which destroys healthy skin tissue, causes most of the skin ageing and wrinkling. Vitamin E is an anti-oxidant and protects cell membranes and other fat-soluble parts of the body from oxidative damage. This can slow down the ageing process of the cells. The polluted air, chlorinated water, ultraviolet rays of the sun, all cause wrinkling and sagging of the skin. Vitamin E nullifies all these harmful and ageing effected through its anti-oxidative properties.

Apart from the skin benefits, the hair loss caused by the oxidation can also be reversed by using vitamin E. Thinning of hair, dryness or damage of hair and dandruff formation are a part of the oxidation process and the anti-oxidative nature of Vitamin E provides a barrier to this process.

Vitamin E can be found in wheat germ, corn, all raw nuts, egg yolk, green leafy vegetables such as spinach and asparagus, and vegetable oils like corn oil, sunflower oil, soyabean oil and cottonseed oil. One can also take supplements of this vitamin if the required level is not available from the natural sources. A daily dose of 100 IU, going up to 400 IU in a gradual manner, should do the trick.

■ ■

Section Two YOUTHFUL FOOD

"On a foundation of good food we can build almost anything. Without it we can build nothing".

—Henry Wallace

Some people may well ask as to what has youth got to do with food. Well, it has all to do with food and nutrition. Food is not just sustenance for some people; it is something that plays a paramount role in tickling the taste buds. There are two kinds of people who inhabit this planet; one who eat to live and the others who live to eat. Needless to say, that the people belonging to the former category are definitely much more healthy than the ones who live by the latter philosophy.

Chapter 1

THE YOUTHFUL DIET

Why do some people look more than their age while others manage to present a youthful picture till they are quite old? In fact, I know a lot many people who do not look half their age. Does it have anything to do with their diet? Of course, it has everything to do with the diet factor.

A person who is young but fat and obese definitely presents an ungainly sight whereas a middle aged but trim person looks more efficient and youthful. Youthful looks don't come with an exercise regimen, alone. Unless an exercise regimen is combined with wise and smart eating, it is of little or no benefit.

Obesity = more input and less output

Fit body = less input and more output

(Input is calories consumed and output is calories expended)

This is a simple formula but makes a lot of sense. Whenever the number of calories consumed by a person is more than the calories expended by him, the extra calories will add up on his body in the form of fat. The only way to get rid of the fat is to begin a diet regimen, which will cut down on the calories consumed even while you work on exercises to increase the calories burnt.

Food Gives Us Energy

Food is the fuel that makes us function, that gives us energy, builds the body and repairs it. Eating is a necessity, but it is also a source of pleasure and a part of our social lives. While in many parts of the world people struggle to eat enough to survive, in affluent countries the culinary delights of food, the domestic routine of mealtimes and other social factors have diverted our eating habits from our real nutritional needs. Hunger, the natural stimulus for eating, has been superseded by habit and custom. The food we eat, far from enhancing our health, is a major contributing factor in serious, widespread health problems, notably heart disease, obesity, cancers, and digestive disorders, the so-called 'diseases of civilisation'.

The rising phenomenon of globalisation along with newfound prosperity in most Indian homes has brought many ills with them. The increased consumption of processed, high-sugar and high-fat foods, foods that were once regarded as luxuries, have brought in many ills to our households.

Changing to a good diet should not be a matter of making stressful adjustments, such as avoiding all sweet and fatty foods, and living on a monotonous fare of brown rice and vegetables. Fad diets are also not the answer either to ill health or to obesity. They can deprive the body of essential nutrients, and lower the body's metabolic rate. What counts most is establishing a good ratio of nutrients, choosing good quality foods, and being aware of special individual requirements. The simplest rule is to choose foods that are as close to their natural state as possible since they are most likely to yield the full range of nutrients that the body needs.

Food Nutrients

An ideal diet is one which provides all the essential elements while cutting out the unnecessary ones. The function of food is to provide energy to sustain the involuntary and voluntary activities necessary for the continuance of life.

The substances in the food on which life depends are the nutrients. Nutrients are the chemical components of food that work in our body. They are required by the body in the right amounts and must be eaten regularly. Balance is the key word in nutrition. A good diet should have the right balance of nutrients. The nutrients that are essential for life and vitality are:

- Carbohydrates • Proteins • Fats • Vitamins
- Minerals • Water • Fibre

Different Elements of A Well Balanced Diet

Carbohydrates

Carbohydrates furnish heat and energy. They are subdivided into three classes – starches, sugars and cellulose. The starches are found in such foods as cereals, breads, macaroni, potatoes, and corn, while the sugars, a more concentrated form of carbohydrate than starches are found in honey, molasses, preserves, dried and fresh fruits, fruit juices, and in cane, beet or maple sugar. Only a small amount of carbohydrates can be stored in the body as such; when taken in excess of body needs, they are changed to fat by the body and stored as fat.

Cellulose is a form of carbohydrate found in fruits, vegetables, and cereals in varying amounts. It is a carbohydrate found in all plants, but human beings do not have the digestive enzyme required to digest this carbohydrate. Nevertheless, cellulose and other indigestible carbohydrates are now thought to be an important part of the diet, as a source of fibre, which aids the passage of material through the bowel.

Proteins

The word 'protein' comes from a Greek verb meaning "to hold first place". Ever since the first uncertain steps were taken in the study of nutrition, scientists have realised the importance of proteins. They are the essential 'building blocks' of the living cells and comprise about 12 per cent of the weight of the human body. Proteins in the food are broken down by digestion into amino acids, which are then rearranged into new proteins needed by the body. If unnecessarily large quantities of protein are eaten, they are used as a source of energy and broken down into simple substances such as carbon dioxide, water and urea, which are excreted in the urine. Amino acids are composed of carbon, hydrogen, oxygen, and nitrogen and sometimes sulphur. Proteins are found to some extent in nearly all foods, since life itself, both plants and animals, cannot exist without them. All necessary protein may be obtained from bread, grains and beans, although meat fish and eggs are good sources.

Fats and Oils

Fats are heat and energy producers in concentrated form, yielding two and a fourth as much energy per ounce as carbohydrates yield. There are many different types of fats and oils. However, the only difference between fats and oil as a whole is that oils are liquid at room temperature. Most animal fats are hard at average room temperatures. Fats can be stored in the body to be used in the future. Since fats contain twice as much energy, weight for weight, as carbohydrates, it is important to cut down on fats when dieting. However, fats and oils are important in cooking because they carry flavours and so they should be mixed judiciously with carbohydrate rich foods.

Vitamins

The vitamins are a group of body regulators, the chemical nature of which is now fairly well established. They are the substances needed by the body, which the body cannot make for itself from raw materials. Vitamins are only needed in small amounts, mostly as catalysts helping along vital chemical reactions. Shortage of vitamins causes deficiency such as scurvy (shortage of vitamin C), rickets (shortage of vitamin D), beri beri (shortage of Vitamin B) and others. A balanced diet contains all the necessary vitamins. It is much more important to try to obtain a good mixed diet, them to attempt to supplement the diet with vitamins. In fact, too much vitamin A or D can be harmful and excess of the others will serve no purpose. However, there are special circumstances, when extra vitamins maybe prescribed by a doctor.

- *Fat-Soluble Vitamins*

They are mainly found in oils and fat-containing foods. Since the body stores these in its fatty tissues, one does not need to eat them every day. Overdoses can be toxic. Vitamins A, D, E and K are Fat-soluble vitamins.

- *Water-Soluble Vitamins*

They are found in a variety of plant and animal foods. Because the body stores them in small amounts and quickly excretes excesses, they need to be part of your diet nearly everyday. Vitamins C and B complex water-soluble vitamins.

Vitamin	Sources	Benefits
Vitamin A (retinal)	Liver (especially fish liver), egg yolk, fortified margarine, oily fish, oranges, apricots, carrots, tomatoes, melons, dark green leafy vegetables.	Needed for maintenance of skin, mucous membranes, bones, teeth and hair, eyesight, and reproduction, may protect against cancer.
Vitamin D (calciferol)	Fortified milk, dairy products, fish liver oils, fatty fish, eggs, and fortified margarine, also synthesized by ultraviolet light.	Helps absorb calcium; needed for bone growth and maintenance.
Vitamin E (tocoferol)	Vegetable oils, nuts, dark green leafy vegetables, whole grain food, wheat germ.	Cell growth, antioxidants
Vitamin K	Most vegetables – especially the dark green leafy ones, eggs, cereals, liver.	Essential in production of some proteins that help in the clotting of blood.
Vitamin B_1 (Thiamine)	Most foods – including wheat germ and pulses, whole grains, brewer's yeast, nuts, fortified breakfast cereals.	Helps break down carbohydrates; nervous system.
Vitamin B_2 (Riboflavin)	Brewer's yeast, liver, milk, kidney, dairy products, wheat bran, wheat germ, eggs.	Repairs body tissues and helps release energy from foods.
Vitamin B_3 (Niacin)	Wheat germ, whole grain cereals, peanuts, legumes, meat and fish.	Essential for tissue chemical reactions, needed for nervous and digestive functions.

Vitamin	Sources	Benefits
Vitamin B_5 (Pantothenic Acid)	Liver, kidney, wholegrain cereals, legumes, eggs, dark green leafy vegetables, milk.	Helps metabolise nutrients.
Vitamin B_6 (Pyridoxine)	Avocados, liver, peanuts, walnuts, pork, poultry, whole grains, egg yolks, lean meat, bananas, fish, potatoes.	Nervous system; skin, red blood cells.
Vitamin B_{12} (Cobalamin)	Liver, kidney, some fish (including shell fish), eggs, milk, milk products.	Healthy blood and nerves.
Vitamin C (Ascorbic acid)	Citrus fruits, potatoes, tomatoes, leafy greens.	Helps heal wounds, may fight colds, flu and infections; protects gums, keeps joints and ligaments in good working order.
Biotin	Liver, eggs, cereals, yeast.	Helps form fatty acids and release energy from carbohydrates and amino acids.
Folacin (folic acid)	Liver, dark green leafy vegetables, orange juice, whole grain breads and cereals, enriched cereals, legumes.	Helps form red blood cells and genetic material.
Choline	Egg yolk, qat, nuts.	Centrolling weight and Cholesterol levels.
Inositol	Wheat, germ, Brewer's yeast, banana liver, brown rice.	Helps to promote cell growth and controls estrogen levels.

Minerals

Minerals are those substances in our food, which furnish building material for bones and teeth, supply valuable constituents to body fluids, and regulate certain body processes. Minerals are found most abundantly in natural, unrefined foods. These minerals are essential for the growth of the body.

• *Minerals essential for the body.*

Mineral	Sources	Essential for
Calcium	Cheese, milk, yoghurt, eggs, bread, nuts, pulses, fish with soft bones such as whitebait and tinned sardines, leafy green vegetables.	Healthy bones, teeth and nails; muscle and nerve function, blood clotting; milk production in nursing mothers.
Chloride	Regulates fluid and electrolyte balances; forms part of gastric juices.	Salt, processed foods.
Magnesium	Needed for bone and teeth formation; aids in release of energy, nerve and muscle function.	Dark green leafy vegetables, nuts, seeds, whole grain foods, legumes, milk.
Phosphorus	Builds and strengthens bones; helps release energy from nutrients.	Milk, cheese, meat, fish, poultry, eggs, whole grains, legumes, nuts.
Potassium	Helps to transmit nerve impulses, control muscle contraction, and maintain proper blood pressure.	Many fruits and vegetables; cereals, legumes, and meat.
Sodium	Regulates fluid and acid base balance.	Salt, processed foods.
Sulphur	Needed to make hair, nails, and cartilage.	Meat, fish, eggs, and legumes.

Some minerals are needed by the body in much smaller amounts, but are no less important for its functioning than the major minerals.

- *Minerals required in smaller amounts.*

Mineral	Benefits	Sources
Chromium	Helps insulin work efficiently in glucose metabolism.	Brewer's yeast, calf's liver, whole-grain cereals, peanuts, wheat germ.
Copper	Needed for iron absorption and metabolism; helps form red blood cells and nerve fibres.	Liver, kidney, seafood, nuts, seeds, tap water.
Fluoride	Contributes to bone and teeth maintenance.	Iodised salt, seafood, saltwater fish, dairy products, and vegetables.
Iodine	Needed to form thyroid hormones.	Iodised salt sea food.
Iron	Liver, red meat, oily fish, whole grain cereals, leafy green vegetables.	Whole grains, fruits, nuts vegetables, tea, legumes.
Manganese	Needed for bone formation, involved in fat synthesis.	Milk, legumes, whole grain breads and cereals.
Molybdenum	Aids in metabolism.	Liver, kidney, seafood, meat and whole grains.
Selenium	Works in association with vitamin E as an antioxidant.	Liver, seafood, meat, eggs, poultry, fish and whole grain cereals.
Zinc	Needed for metabolism and digestion; aids in wound healing, growth, tissue repair, and sexual development.	Liver, seafood, beans, whole grain cereals, nuts.

Water

Not enough attention has been paid to water and its importance in diet. Water is one of the most necessary elements for our body to operate efficiently. Every cell in our body depends upon water to function properly yet most of us do not understand the role of this vital nutrient.

It takes just two atoms of hydrogen and one atom of oxygen to create the unique essence of human life...water. The power of this thirst quencher, skin purifier, stomach cleanser, weight controller and cornucopia of good health has often been underestimated.

Up to 70 per cent of our total body weight comes from water. Inadequate intake of water could lead to major diseases that modern medicine can treat but fail to cure. Along with being a natural curative, a sip of water lowers body temperature, dilutes blood to the required consistency, promotes excretion of poisons from the skin in the form of evaporation, stimulates the normal functions of the kidneys and increases the movements of the intestines. Hot water works as a laxative and sedative and relieves pain, cramps and spasms. It also increases the metabolic rate and aids digestion.

Water acts as a solvent, coolant, lubricant and transport agent. The amount of body water varies with body fat. The percentage of water to body weight is greater in lean individuals. This is due to the nearly water free characteristics of fat tissue, which results in bodies with more fatty tissues containing proportionately less water than bodies with less fatty tissue.

Besides keeping body temperature stable, water carries nutrients, eliminates toxins and waste products, maintains blood volume and provides the medium in which chemical reactions occur in the cells.

The body has three sources of water: fluid intake, water content of food, and the fluid released during metabolism of proteins, carbohydrates and lipids.

Though thirst is the body's way of signalling that water is required, most of us ignore the signal. Most people, on average, drink only eight ounces (one cup) of water per day as against the recommended intake of at least 6-8 glasses per day. The rest of the water the body needs must be extracted from other liquids or foods that we eat. Not enough water is a real threat to the system. Many chemical reactions inside the body will not occur without the right amount of water.

A small change makes a big difference when it comes to water. If you do a lot of travel by air, you can lose as much as two pounds of water in a three to four hour flight. Stress, alcohol and caffeine all influence the amount of water and the speed in which your body loses it. Any of these factors, alone or in combination, could cause a small but critical shrinkage of the brain. This small shrinkage will impair neuromuscular coordination, decrease concentration, and slow down thinking. The average amount of water loss per day is two cups through breathing, two cups through invisible perspiration, and six cups through urination and bowel movements. That is a total of ten cups lost per day without taking into account perspiration from exercise or hard work, excessively dry air, or alcohol and caffeine consumption.

Fibre

Also known as roughage, fibre is a component of food that is more or less indigestible and can be found in all fruits, vegetables and whole grains. Fibres can be either insoluble (the less digestible bran fibre) or soluble (cellulose fibres from fruits and vegetables). For good health, you need both types of fibres in your diet.

Fibre is important to your body because it helps with the proper functioning of the intestinal tract as it speeds the elimination of waste products. It is a natural laxative and alleviates constipation. Those suffering from constipation should have a rich fibre diet. In addition, a rich fibre diet prevents against colon cancer, as there is less exposure of cancer causing agents to the intestinal tract.

Individuals with diabetes may also benefit from a high fibre diet since it modulates the rate at which glucose enters the blood and prevents increases in blood levels of sugar and insulin. Soluble fibre may also help to reduce cholesterol levels. Because fibre is filling, it provides a sense of satiety with far fewer calories than fat, thus controlling obesity and hypertension. A research done by the US-based Nurses Health Study found that the risk of heart attack was significantly lower among women who consumed an average of 23 grams of fibre.

Sources of fibre – Whole grain bread and cereals; raw fruits and berries such as apples, plums, cherries, grapes, oranges, bananas, apricots, strawberries, raisins and dried fruits and vegetables such as beans, cabbage, carrot, cauliflower, celery cucumber, lettuce, onions and spinach. However, increase the fibre in your diet slowly to prevent abdominal bloating, gas and flatulence.

Ten Commandments of Weight Loss

Losing weight can be confusing, but if you start to incorporate the 10 Commandments of Weight Loss into your everyday life, you will soon see big changes in the way you look and feel.

1. ***Eat less fat:*** Keep your fat intake less than 30 percent of your total calories. One gram of fat contains nine calories. If you cut back on fat, you'll control your weight, lower your risk of heart disease and boost your energy. Try replacing high-fat foods with nutritious low-fat options like fruits, veggies and grains, rather than processed, sugary, fat-free snacks that are nutritional zeros.
2. ***Eat less saturated fat:*** Saturated fat clogs your arteries by increasing your cholesterol levels even more than cholesterol does. Keep saturated fat to less than 10 percent of your total calories. If you eat 2,000 calories per day, try to eat less than 22 grams of saturated fat. Beef, whole milk and cheese are all loaded with saturated fats. Replace them with lower fat cuts of meat, skim milk and cut down on the cheese.
3. ***Watch your portions:*** One theory why the waistlines continue to expand is because portion sizes keep growing. Restaurants serve mammoth-size meals, and we have become accustomed to eating bigger meals and snacks. By simply cutting back on portions sizes you will be cutting back on calories.
4. ***Combine carbohydrates and protein in meals and snacks:*** Don't believe the myth that you shouldn't combine protein and carbohydrates in the same meal. These macronutrients work great together. Carbohydrates tend to give you an immediate energy boost, but the effect wears off quickly and you soon feel tired or hungry (think about how you feel after eating just a sandwich). Protein-rich foods can neutralise those feelings, keeping you alert and feeling full much longer. So instead of just having a sandwich and juice for breakfast, include some low-fat yoghurt or add some peanut butter or low-fat cream cheese to your sandwich.

5. ***Drink up:*** Water is one of the most important nutrients for your body. It cushions your organs, lubricates your joints, and keeps your skin looking good. Even a tiny water deficit can radically affect how your body and mind perform. You need to drink at least 8-10 glasses of water a day.

   Be sure to drink before, during and after every workout. Don't wait until you're thirsty to drink—that's a telltale sign that you're already dehydrated. Instead, you need to check your urine. You should be urinating every two to four hours throughout the day. It should be clear to pale yellow.

6. ***Build up your bones:*** You may think you don't have to worry about your bones now, but if you don't, you will definitely need to worry about them down the road. There are two proven methods for keeping bones strong and preventing osteoporosis: Get enough calcium and pump iron. Experts recommend getting at least 1,000 milligrams of calcium per day (twice as much as the average woman takes in), and some say that 1,500 milligrams is optimal. One cup of plain low-fat yoghurt has about 400 milligrams of calcium; a cup of skim milk has about 300 milligrams; and three ounces of salmon has about 370 milligrams. Other calcium-rich sources include green veggies, such as leafy greens, kale, spinach and broccoli.

7. ***Eat early and often:*** To keep from running on empty and help you control your weight, try eating four to six meals a day. Start first thing in the morning (after a seven or eight hour fast, you need to eat). Without breakfast your body has no fuel to function, and your brain and body are left running on fumes.

   Limiting your food intake to the traditional three-meals-a-day can cause wide swings in your blood sugar levels, which can also affect your energy and moods. Baby yourself when it comes to meals and snacks. What keeps most babies happy and cranky-free? Being fed continuously through the day. Eating throughout the day is also a great weight-loss strategy. If you're never too hungry, tired or cranky, you're much less likely reach for a Kit Kat bar. Eating large meals may also make you feel sluggish and groggy, because your body needs to shift extra blood from your brain to your belly to digest the food. Meals that weigh in at over 1,000 calories are not a good idea in the middle of the day or before you work out.

8. ***Variety is the spice of life:*** Varying the foods you eat will keep your diet nutrient-rich and your taste buds from getting bored. Studies show that tired taste buds lead to overeating. Keep them busy enjoying a wide variety of foods. Most people eat only 20 to 25 different foods, which strictly limit the nutrients you get. Even if you're getting a healthy balance of vitamins and minerals, you may be missing out on hundreds—if not thousands—of phytochemicals (substances in grains, fruits and veggies that appear to have important cancer-fighting properties). One simple way to add nutrients and wake up your taste buds is to try a new food every month.

9. ***Eat more fruits and vegetables:*** You may be tired of hearing that you should eat more fruits and veggies, but if you want to lose weight, they are a great calorie-bargain. People who have been successful at maintaining weight loss tend to eat more fruits and veggies than the average person. They're a key source of fibre, and they contain a wealth of cancer-fighting vitamins, mineral and phytochemicals. A diet high in fruits and vegetables can significantly cut the risk of cancers of the lung, colon, pancreas, stomach, bladder and ovaries.

   Stick to whole fruits rather than processed juices; a large apple, for instance, has four grams of fibre, whereas a cup of apple juice contains none. Whether you are interested in weight loss or simply want to maintain your weight and stay healthy, set your fruits and veggies goal at five servings a day.

10. ***Eat more fibre:*** Fibre not only keeps you regular and help prevent certain diseases, but it can help you lose weight too. Fibre-packed foods (beans, grains, fruits and vegetables) tend to be low in fat and rich in vitamins, and they make you feel full! Insoluble fibres (found in bran, whole-grain breads, cereals and fruits) reduce constipation and may lower your risk of colon cancer. Soluble fibres (apples, citrus fruits, oats and cooked dried beans) may reduce heart-disease risk by keeping blood cholesterol levels low. Adults need to eat 25 to 35 grams of fibres daily.

■■

Chapter 2

VEGETARIANISM

Vegetarians are people who do not eat meat products and may also not consume dairy products or eggs. They may do so for health reasons or for philosophical and moral reasons. Some people, such as Jains and Brahmins are vegetarians because of their religious beliefs.

There are three main types of vegetarians: lacto-ovo-vegetarians, who eat dairy foods and eggs; lacto-vegetarians, who eat dairy foods, but no eggs; and vegans who consume no animal foods of any type.

Food influences every aspect of our well being including the physical and emotional well-being. There are arguments for and against vegetarian diet. Many argue that man was born to be a vegetarian and God intended him to be so, it is only a deviation of that fact that we have taken to eating non-vegetarian food. The feeling that if nature wanted us to be meat eaters, she would have equipped us with sharp pointed teeth to tear into the flesh and acidic saliva to digest the animal protein backs their theory. For instance, carnivorous animals have claws, teeth that can tear into flesh and round stomach, which produce enough hydrochloric acid to digest meat. They also have shorter intestinal length to shorten the process of meat digestion and a liver that is equipped to get rid of excess uric acid.

That man was created as a vegetarian is borne out by the molars that are designed to crush and grind. Our saliva is alkaline in nature, which is perfect to digest plant protein; we have a stomach and greater length of intestine, designed for vegetarian food. The liver of human beings is also not equipped with the capacity of getting rid of the excess uric acid that the animal protein break down produces. That is one of the prime reasons for the painful disease called gout.

On the other hand, the proponents of non-vegetarianism argue that all food that can be digested by man should be considered normal and healthy. Their point is that only non-vegetarian food can provide all the elements of a nutritious diet and so it is healthier than the vegan diet.

There are many factors against the consumption of meat. Animal protein is tough to digest and the food putrefies inside the system creating toxins that are harmful to the body.

The Ayurvedic Theory

According to ayurveda, there are positive and negative attributes of diet. Since ayurveda deals with a holistic approach to healing, it covers the diet factor in depth.

Ayurveda has categorised personality traits into three different kinds, based on the food we eat– the *Satvik* or the spiritual quality, *Rajasik* or active quality, and *Tamasik* or material quality of the mind are all affected by the food we eat. The activating *Rajasik* quality may dominate or combine with the other two qualities to form different mental tendencies in man; spiritually active, intellectually active, or materially active.

Satvik food is food that can be 'digested easily' and has the quality of bringing a balance to one's mind. It helps in building immunity and improving the healing response in those who are unwell. *Satvik* food is all food that is closest to their natural form and includes milk, milk products, fruits, most fresh vegetables expect the ones that belong to the onion family like garlic, onion, scallions, and chives.

Whole grain cereals like most lentils, sprouts and natural sweeteners like jaggery, honey are also included in *Satvik* diet. Also included in this category are the natural oils like ghee, butter and vegetable oils.

Satvik food is moderately cooked with few spices and less fat. Chillies and black pepper are not used in cooking. Common spices like turmeric, ginger, cinnamon, coriander, aniseed and cardamom are, however, used in *Satvik* cooking. Eating raw foods is not considered *Satvik* as they harbour a lot of parasites and microbes. According to ayurveda, raw foods are known to weaken the digestive system and reduce '*ojas*' which is synonymous with vital energy also known as '*prana*'. Prana is also known as 'Chi' and 'Qi' or 'jing'. Simplified, it means the life force.

The proper functioning of the mind and spiritual development depend on ojas. A person who follows the Satvik food habits is known to possess a clear mind, is balanced, moderate in habits and a focussed person. He usually avoids using intoxicants like alcohol, stimulants like tea, coffee, tobacco and non-vegetarian food. A Satvik person is also supposed to be spiritually aware and extremely balanced.

Rajasik food is food, which is fresh but 'heavy' to digest. Those who indulge in heavy physical activity should eat this type of food. It includes non-vegetarian food like meat, fish, eggs, chicken, all whole pulses and dals, which are not sprouted. Hot spices like chillies, pepper, vegetables including onions and garlic are all included under this category. The *Rajasik* food is cooked fresh as in *Satvik* cooking, and is of high quality and nutrient density. It also contains more spices and oil than *Satvik* cooking.

This kind of food is known to make a person long for sensual stimulation. He is usually aggressive in nature in a positive way and is of energetic disposition. He is interested in power, prestige, position and prosperity. But he is in control of his life and not obsessed by the power and position. A *Rajasik* personality loves to enjoy life.

Tamasik food includes all kinds of food that are not fresh and are unnatural, overcooked, stale and processed. All foods made from refined flour, pastries, pizzas, burgers, chocolates, soft drinks, stimulants like tea, coffee, tobacco, intoxicants like alcohol and wines fall under the *Tamasik* category. Even the canned and preserved foods like jams, jellies, pickles and fermented food come under this group. Fried foods, sweets made from sugar, ice creams, pudding and most modern day junk foods, all kinds of spicy, salty, sweet, and fatty foods are also included in this list.

The *Tamasik* people usually lead a sedentary lifestyle and enjoy packaged and processed foods, which are rich in calories. They have no control over their tongue and indulge in mindless eating. Such individuals would benefit from switching from a *Tamasik* diet into a *Satvik* one.

The bane of today's generation is that they are the *Tamasik* personalities. Self centred, insecure and ailing, they are reaching a point of no return. The very food that has become a status symbol and an epitome of fashion is of unhealthy nature. We are leaving the wisdom of *Satvik* food and rushing towards the ills of an unhealthy *Tamasik* diet. No wonder our society is degenerating into a violent, self-seeking, power hungry and uncaring one.

Benefits of Vegetarianism

Since vegetarian diets are low in animal products they are typically lower than non-vegetarian diets in total fat, saturated fat, and cholesterol. These factors are associated with increased risk of obesity, coronary heart disease (which causes heart attack), high blood pressure, diabetes mellitus, and some forms of cancer. Thus, it is logical that vegetarian diets are healthful and nutritionally adequate when appropriately planned.

Vegetarians have lower average blood cholesterol and therefore have a reduced risk of coronary artery disease. They have a lower risk of obesity and suffer from fewer digestive problems when compared to non-vegetarians.

Plant foods have been shown to have "chemo-preventive" properties. Risk of lung cancer in heavy smokers has been shown to be reduced in populations eating generous amounts of plant foods, and risk of breast, prostate and other cancers is substantially lower in populations, which consume vegetarian or largely vegetarian diets.

Researchers have identified eight food groups, each of which has unique cancer-preventing qualities. All eight of the food groups come from the plant kingdom. Conversely, animal product consumption is implicated in a host of degenerative diseases including cancer and heart disease, and animal-source foods in general provide little or no protection against most health conditions other than starvation.

Combining Foods for Balanced Nutrition

Vegans must plan their diet especially well because no single fruit, vegetable or grain contains the nutritionally complete protein food that is found in meat, milk and eggs. Beans, nuts, peas and many other vegetarian foods contain large amounts of protein. However, these foods must be eaten in particular combinations to provide the body with nutritionally complete protein. For example, beans and rice eaten together provide complete protein, but neither food does this when eaten in isolation.

To obtain calcium, vegans must eat sesame seeds or certain green leafy vegetables, such as broccoli or spinach. The iron and other elements in these vegetables are absorbed better when combined with vitamin C so squeezing a lime on the dish makes it easier to absorb the nutrients.

Soya Goodness

For thousands of years, populations throughout much of the world consumed soybeans without realising that this bean has some miraculous health properties. The Chinese and Japanese cuisine is replete with recipes that incorporate this wonder food.

Today, soya has become the centre of a lot of attention. Researchers are studying the compounds found in soy that may not only help reduce the risk of some diseases, such as heart disease, osteoporosis and cancer, but also help alleviate the symptoms of menopause. Doctors found that when animal protein coming from meat was replaced by textured soyabean protein in patients suffering with elevated blood cholesterol, there was a significant reduction in blood cholesterol levels. Further research discovered that the protein from soyabeans contains a unique amino acid composition, which seems to produce the cholesterol lowering effect.

For vegetarians, this food takes on a special relevance since it compensates for the nutritional loss of a vegetarian diet.

Listed below are some of the more common soya foods in the market today.

Green vegetable soyabeans (edamamé)

These large soyabeans are harvested when the beans are still green and taste sweet. They can be served as a snack or a main vegetable dish, after boiling in slightly salted water for 15 to 20 minutes. They are high in protein and fibre and contain no cholesterol.

Meat alternatives (meat analogs)

Meat alternatives (also called meat analogs) are non-meat foods made from soya protein and other ingredients mixed together to simulate various kinds of meat. Usually, they can be used the same way as the foods they replace. .

Soya cheese

Soya cheese is made from soyamilk. It can substitute for sour cream or cream cheese and can be found in variety of flavours in natural-food stores.

Soya flour

Soya flour is made from roasted soyabeans that are ground into a fine powder. To turn normal wheat flour into protein packed one, mix in soyaflour which can easily be made out of soyabean. Soya flour is gluten-free, so yeast-raised breads made with soya flour are more dense in texture. Replace ¼ to 1/3 of the flour called for in a recipe (for muffins, cakes, cookies, pancakes and quick breads) with soya flour.

Soya granules

Soya granules are similar to soya flour, except that the soyabeans have been toasted and cracked into coarse pieces, rather than the fine powder of soya flour. Soya grits can be used as a substitute for flour in some recipes. High in protein, soya grits can be cooked together with other grains.

Soya protein isolates (isolated soya protein)

When protein is removed from defatted flakes, the result is soya protein isolates. Soya protein isolates contain the most amount of protein of all soya products.

Textured soya flour (TSF)

Running defatted soya flour through an extrusion cooker, which allows for many different forms and sizes, makes TSF. When hydrated, it has a chewy texture. It is widely used as a meat extender. Textured soya flour contains about 70 percent protein and retains most of the bean's dietary fibre. Often referred to simply as textured soya protein (TSP), textured soya flour is sold dried in granular and chunk style.

Soya sauce

Soya sauce is a dark brown liquid made from soyabeans that have undergone a fermenting process. Soya sauces have a salty taste, but are lower in sodium than traditional table salt. Soya sauce is extensively used in Chinese cuisine.

Soya yoghurt

Soya yoghurt is made from soyamilk. Its creamy texture makes it an easy substitute for sour cream or cream cheese. Soya yoghurt can be found in variety of flavours in natural-food stores.

Soyabeans, whole

As soyabeans mature in the pod, they ripen into a hard, dry bean. Most soyabeans are yellow, but there are brown and black varieties. Whole soyabeans (an excellent source of protein and dietary fibre) can be cooked and used in sauces, stews and soups. Whole soyabeans that have been soaked can be roasted for snacks.

Soya milk, soya beverages

Soyabeans, soaked, ground fine and strained, produce a fluid called soybean milk, which is a good substitute for cow's milk. Plain, unfortified soya milk is an excellent source of high-quality protein and B-vitamins.

Soya nuts

Roasted soya nuts are whole soyabeans that have been soaked in water and then baked until browned. Soya nuts can be found in a variety of flavours, including chocolate. High in protein and isoflavones, soy nuts are similar in texture and flavour to peanuts.

Soya oil and products

Soya oil is the natural oil extracted from whole soyabeans. Oil sold in the grocery store under the generic name "vegetable oil" is usually 100 percent soya oil or a blend of soya oil and other oils. Read the label to make certain you are buying soyabean oil. Soya oil is cholesterol-free and high in polyunsaturated fat. Soya oil also is used to make margarine and shortening.

Tofu and tofu products

Tofu, also known as soyabean curd, is a soft cheese-like food made by curdling fresh, hot soymilk with a coagulant. Tofu is a bland product that easily absorbs the flavours of other ingredients with which it is cooked. Tofu is rich in high-quality protein and B-vitamins and is low in sodium.

Firm tofu (easy to stir fry or grill) is dense and solid and can be cubed and served in soups. Firm tofu is higher in protein, fat and calcium than other forms of tofu. Soft tofu is good for recipes that call for blended tofu. Silken tofu is a creamy product and can be used as a replacement for sour cream in many dip recipes.

A good diet can also be an interesting and tasty one, provided one can be creative about putting it together. All one needs to remember is that we should not become slaves to our taste buds, which may learn to appreciate the rich and spicy stuff more than the nutritious one. Imaginative experimentation with various food combinations and learning the art of calorie balancing could work wonders with one's fitness and health.

Tips for Vegetarians

- Vegetarian diets of any type should include a wide variety of foods and enough calories to meet your energy needs.
- Keep your intake of sweets and fatty foods to a minimum. These foods are low in nutrient density.
- Choose whole or unrefined grain products when possible, or use fortified or enriched cereal products.
- Use a variety of fruits and vegetables, including foods that are good sources of vitamins A and C.
- If you use milk or dairy products, choose skim or low-fat or non-fat varieties.
- Eggs are considered alright for most vegetarian diets, but one must use it with moderation. Because eggs have a high cholesterol content (213 mg per yolk), monitor your use of eggs as you try to limit your cholesterol intake to no more than 300 mg per day.

■ ■

Chapter 3

DAMAGING FOODS

In different parts of the world, people's bodies have adapted, over hundreds of years, to a variety of diets. But the alterations in the diet have been so rapid that the body has been unable to adjust fast enough. For example, the intake of sugar has increased many folds over the past three to four decades. The consumption of fats, food additives, soft drinks, refined and processed foods have increased to unhealthy proportions. Most of the good value foods are now on the wane in many households, instead fast foods have replaced the menu. Eating out has become another trend, which is neither healthy nor economical.

Most people heap their systems with unhealthy food, which causes a lot of harm. Some of the damaging food habits become so addicting that people do not like giving them up or settling for something as insipid as a vegetable juice.

Sugar

Refined sugar supplies only 'empty' calories, i.e. no nutrients, only energy. It is the major cause of tooth decay and it is a principal factor in diabetes, obesity, and certain other disorders. It makes us hungry by creating a 'roller coaster' effect in our blood sugar levels: blood sugar soars, the pancreas reacts by secreting more insulin, then levels rapidly plummet, making us tired, hungry and depressed. This is the low blood sugar syndrome hypoglycaemia.

We do need sugar as a vital source of fuel. The best source is from natural sources in whole foods, where they are balanced with the proper minerals. Processed white sugar has all the minerals and vitamins removed. Read all labels carefully as most canned/processed foods contain sugar. Sugar often appears as sucrose, dextrose, glucose, corn sweetener, corn syrup, high fructose corn syrup and maltose. It's in salad dressing, cereals, energy bars and foods that you least suspect.

Refined sugar passes quickly into the blood stream and shocks the stomach and pancreas. It causes an acidic condition in the body and the body rushes to neutralise this using its reserves of minerals to do so. Calcium is one of these and is used up quickly. Calcium is one of the essential nutrients used in the contraction of muscle fibres. A muscle cannot relax without proper amounts of calcium.

Over time, conditions of hypoglycaemia and diabetes can result from constant intake of sugar. The adrenal glands also become stressed, resulting in conditions of fatigue and impaired immune function. Sugar contributes to mental clarity, ADD, arteriosclerosis, anxiety, irritability, shakiness, headaches, insomnia and many more symptoms and conditions.

What should you do: Balance your meals with more protein to help reduce sugar cravings.

There are also many supplements to help ease the addiction. Some that have been found to work are chromium picolinate, biotin, and vitamins B complex and C.

Caffeine

Caffeine is actually a drug and it is addicting. Caffeine produces an initial surge of energy, alertness, and well being through its direct effect on the nervous system and adrenal glands. With this constant stimulation the nervous system and adrenal glands become stressed and overworked causing fatigue and immune system problems in the long run. This stimulant also activates the contraction of muscles adding to tightness that may already be there.

Coffee and caffeine-rich foods, like chocolate, tea, and cola drinks, produced a release of the body's stored sugar to combat the influx of what is essentially a poison. Like alcohol it provokes hypertension and nervous symptoms. Cholesterol levels go up and B vitamins and some minerals are depleted. Excess caffeine may also be involved in breast and prostate problems.

Coffee beans are the most known source of caffeine. They are grown with the use of pesticides and herbicides that are toxic in nature. Caffeine is also found in chocolate, cola's and other soft drinks and some over the counter drugs such as Excedrin and Anacin. Some signs of caffeine problems are fatigue, headache, depression, insomnia, anxiety, muscle tightness, high blood pressure and PMS.

People suffering from insomnia will realise that their sleep improves after stopping that coffee before bedtime. Coffee and tea are known to stimulate gastric secretion. Patients with peptic ulcer should restrict their use. They should drink fewer cups and add more milk or cream to their beverage. Heart patients and those with high blood pressure should also avoid or reduce the frequency and strength of their drink because caffeine stimulates cardiac muscles, increases the cardiac output, has deleterious effect on blood vessels.

Cerebral vessels are constricted by caffeine. There is a risk of an increase in blood pressure if tea or coffee is taken in excess. Expectant mothers and those breast-feeding should cut down on their coffee. The caffeine in the coffee drunk by the mother is ingested by the foetus in the womb and by the suckling child through breast milk. The infant has no means of breaking down the components of the same and hence accumulates it in his body system. Drinking of coffee is also harmful to the pancreas. It may lead to pancreatic cancer.

If you get a headache when you don't have your morning coffee, you are addicted to this drug. Gradually ending the intake of this substance is recommended. Begin with cutting back on the daily amount and substitute with other products such as teas and coffee substitutes.

Caffeine Levels

The caffeine content of a cup of coffee depends on the type of bean and how it was processed and brewed. Tea's caffeine content increases the longer it steeps.

Item	Caffeine (mg)
Coffee (1 cup)	
Regular, drip	60-180
Regular, percolated	40-170
Regular, instant	30-120
Decaffeinated, brewed	2-5
Decaffeinated, instant	1-5
Tea (1 cup)	
Brewed	25-110
Instant	25-50
Cola drinks and chocolate	
Cola drinks (1 bottle)	30-60
Chocolate milk (250 ml)	2-7
Cocoa (1 cup)	2-20

Soft Drinks

Soft drinks are bad for health due to the same caffeine factor and sugar content.

Eliminate the intake of soft drinks substituting with water with lemon or herbal teas. Drinking synthetic cold drinks has become a fad. The high amount of money spent in advertising these drinks has also boosted the sales and popularity of the soft drinks. These contain gas and synthetic colours, which may look very attractive, but actually contain toxic substances. Carbon dioxide is a gas we breathe out. Through these cold drinks, we are breathing this gas in again, and our body will have to spend some energy in breathing it out.

Animal Protein

Although animal flesh, eggs, dairy produce, etc. provide the complete protein that is necessary to health, in excess it can be harmful. People who live on a high animal protein diet are thought to be more disposed to bowel cancer, hypertension, diverticulosis and atherosclerosis.

Animal fats are saturated fats and bring about free radical formation to some extent. They not only enhance ageing but also hasten the onset of diseases like cancer of the colon and breast. Most popular sources of animal fats like Cheese, full fat milk, ghee, red meat, beef, skin of chicken etc. can cause a lot of damage to the health.

Excessive intake of red meat also stimulates calcium loss, and reduces bone density leading to osteoporosis. Instead, eating white meat like chicken and turkey is better than eating red meat. However, do not eat the skin of chicken since it has high fat content.

The animal protein component in food should be cut down, especially as one grows in age. It is a misconception that only non-vegetarian food provides complete protein. Vegetarian foods can also provide all the protein elements when they are properly combined. In fact, more and more people are turning to vegetarianism because of the benefits it provides.

Refined Foods

The inevitable result of a diet high in refined starches is a decrease in the consumption of fibre. Without fibre, food can take up to 70-80 hours to pass through the digestive tract. Lack of fibre in the diet is responsible for sluggish bowels, constipation and more serious disorders such as diverticulosis and possible cancer of the colon. A whole food diet, with plenty of fresh vegetables and fruits, provides sufficient fibre.

Additives

To enhance the flavour and appearance of processed and packaged foods, and to ensure a long shelf life in the shops, food manufacturers add a wide range of chemicals to their products. Over 3,000 are currently used. A large number have been removed from the 'permitted' list, but the long-term effects of those that remain have not yet been fully evaluated. Additives have been blamed for hyperactivity in children, for decalcification of the bone, and for some types of cancers, too. Meat, fruit and vegetables may have unwanted ingredients like residues of artificial fertilizers and pesticides, and hormones and antibodies given to animals. The accumulation of these toxic compounds in our systems can have a lethal effect on our health and well-being.

Eggs

Eggs have been held responsible for the increase of cholesterol in the body. Too many eggs can be quite harmful but if one removes the yolk, the harmful effect can be controlled to a large extent. The benefits are that an egg is rich source of nutrients so it should not be completely cut out of the diet. Restricting the intake to about 4-5 per week should work fine and if the yolk is removed, the number could go up to 7 per week.

The Egg Yolk

It contains proteins and is rich in fat-soluble vitamins as well as minerals like phosphorus, calcium and iron. An average egg contains 100 mg of cholesterol and that is what makes it dangerous for the middle-aged people.

Saturated Fats

Excess saturated fats have been implicated in cancers, obesity, cardiac disease, and a host of other disorders. Too much saturated fat makes too much cholesterol, which may build up on the arterial walls, from childhood onwards, resulting in atherosclerosis (hardened arteries from fatty deposits). All the fried food that goes under the label of gourmet food and attracts hordes of eager diners to the high-flying restaurants helps the consumption of an unhealthy amount of saturated fats. Bland food, which has less of oil and spices, is hardly palatable to the adventurous tongue and so people flock to the eateries that cater to the rich and spicy favourites. The result is an increased intake of fats.

Dairy products and fatty meats are major culprits; wild game has more polyunsaturated fat, and contains a substance that is thought to protect against atherosclerosis.

Fats that we eat are made up of two chemicals: fatty acid and glycerol. These are formed from carbon, hydrogen and oxygen. These can be either saturated or unsaturated depending on the structure of the fatty acids. The more hydrogen atoms a fatty acid has, the more saturated it is. The degree of fatty acid saturation varies widely.

Body Uses Fats

Fats are part of the wall surrounding every body cell. Fats in small amounts are essential and perform some pretty vital jobs. They insulate the body against cold, serve as a reserve store of energy, act as shock absorbers around the bones and organs, insulate nerve cables, lubricate the skin and help transport certain essential vitamins.

Harmful Effects of Fat

The excess fat is stored in body cells making you overweight. By consuming fats/oils that are easily oxidisable, you predispose your body to the risk of free radical formation. These free radicals make the body cells diseased and dysfunctional. Besides the medical repercussions such as stroke, heart ailments, etc., this excess fat also accelerates ageing. The type of fat you take in is the key to how fast you age.

Good Fat and Bad Fat

Cholesterol rich foods such as egg, red meat, butter and cheese are oxidised easily and promote premature ageing. This type of fats ruins the arteries by elevating the bad cholesterol or the low-density level (LDL) cholesterol. They oxidise the LDL cholesterol, which can then penetrate the artery walls thereby clogging them and increasing the possibility of heart attack. On the other hand, mono-unsaturated fats are slow to oxidise and hence don't cause cell damage. They include olive oil, almond oil, walnut oil, fish oils, flaxseed oil, etc.

Animal fats like butter and ghee increase the production of inflammatory agents in the body causing arthritis, choking of arteries, migraine and some skin problems. All these are also considered the manifestations of ageing.

The Right Choice

- Switch to olive oil.
- Use olive oil for cooking and as salad dressings. Research has shown that consuming, at least, two tablespoons of olive oil can cut the risk of breast cancer by about thirty percent. Moreover, like the other mono-unsaturates, it also selectively lowers the (LDLs bad) leaving the (good) HDLs intact.

- Use minimum quantity of other oil.
- Using 2-3 tsp. of other oils daily is just enough for the necessary body function.

Cooking with Oils

Corn oil – although corn oil is healthy, this is the least satisfactory of the recommended vegetable oils for cooking purposes. For salads, the flavour is rather powerful. If you do not find the flavour attractive, try mixing in some olive oil for cooking or salads.

Olive oil – Olive oil is delicious and can be used for everything, but it is expensive. It has a lovely fruity flavour, which varies tremendously from country to country. However, it is wasteful to use this oil for frying, since it loses its delicious flavour at high temperatures. Use it for rubbing on to meat or fish before grilling, for marinades, for lubricating freshly cooked pasta, and of course for all salads.

Salad oil – mixing four tablespoons of sunflower oil with two dessertspoons of walnut oil, which has a delicious flavour, makes an interesting salad oil.

Soya oil – Soya oil is good for frying, but it starts to taste and smell a bit strong at high temperatures. It has the right consistency for salads. This is the oil used in Japan, where they have so little heart disease. Nutritionally, it is a highly recommended oil.

Sunflower oil – the sunflower oil is excellent for frying as it is almost tasteless and does not smell. It gives a very crisp result. As it is so light and thin it makes a rather dull salad dressing. It is the most versatile of the recommended poly-unsaturated oils but it is expensive.

Say 'No' to Hydrogenated Oils

Never use hydrogenated oils because they increase the risk of heart disease and also produce more free radicals in the body, which in turn advance ageing.

Salt

Common table salt, known chemically as sodium chloride, is the main source of sodium in our diets. Sodium is an essential nutrient required by the body to help regulate its fluid balance, maintain heart rhythm, conduct nerve impulses, and contract muscles. For body requirement, a safe minimum is 500 milligrams of sodium, about a quarter teaspoon of table salt is enough. Most people consume about twice the daily maximum (3000 milligram of sodium – about teaspoon and a half of table salt) recommended by doctors.

The common belief is that the blood pressure rises with age. Expected blood pressure is usually expressed as "100 plus your age". This holds true for many individuals but it is not normal. In fact, blood pressure does not rise with age in everyone, although a large proportion of people – 15% of young adults and 40% of elderly – have high blood pressure.

In certain societies blood pressure does not rise with age and hypertension does not occur. These societies include Pacific Islanders, South American Indians and Aboriginal tribes people. And there are others, all of who live in harmony with their natural environment. They eat a variety of vegetables and fruits and freshly prepared, unsalted food, so the amount of sodium in their diet is a small proportion of what we eat. This is an important difference, which could account for the differences in blood pressure between them and us.

Reduction of sodium intake to 1 millimole per kilogram of ideal body weight will lower blood pressure in those with hypertension. In others, it will prevent hypertension from too much sodium. If sodium intake is reduced while people are young, the rise in blood pressure with age could be prevented.

The relationship between salt intake and hypertension (high blood pressure) is complex and not fully understood but the direct relationship between sodium consumption and the high incidence of high blood pressure has been demonstrated in a number of studies. About 10-15 percent of people are actually 'sodium-sensitive' meaning that consuming too much salt directly elevates their blood pressure.

Healthy adults should reduce their sodium intake to no more than 2400 milligrams per day. This is about 1¼ teaspoons of sodium chloride (salt). To illustrate, the following are sources of sodium in the diet.

1 teaspoon salt = 2000 mg sodium

1 teaspoon baking soda = 1000 mg sodium

These are two major sources of sodium in the foods we eat. It is present in raw foods but the major source is salt, which is added during manufacture and preparation of food.

Normal Sodium Requirement

The amount of sodium required will depend on ideal body weight and is equivalent to 1 mmol per kilogram, per day. A man who, for example, is 176 cm tall and weighs 70 kg is at ideal body weight. Therefore, his recommended dietary sodium intake is 70 mmol of sodium per day. Ten mmols (millimoles) or meq (milli-equivalents) of sodium is contained in 0.58 grams of sodium chloride. Sodium makes up 40% of sodium chloride by weight.

Infants require less sodium (10-49 mmols a day) than adults. Sufficient sodium to meet baby's needs is present in breast milk even though, when compared with cow's milk, breast milk has only one-third amount of sodium. Older children up to their teens will need a slightly higher sodium intake per body weight than adults but this will be obtained if food intake is adequate to maintain growth and ideal body weight.

Sources of Salt

There are many hidden sources of salt. One of the main sources of sodium in the diet is the group of staple items – bread, butter or margarine and cheese. Breads generally contain salt and so do biscuits. Cheeses are very high in salt, too. Apart from these most of the processed foods like gravy powder, stock cubes, yeast extracts, peanut butter, pickles and olives also contain sodium.

Some minor sources of sodium in our diet are mineral replacement drinks, mega doses of vitamin C and some soluble painkillers.

The natural sodium content of fresh foods does not really present a problem because it is relatively low in most foods. Some seafoods are among the exception. Prawns and scallops, for example, have significant sodium content but these do not usually form a large part of most people's diet.

Protein foods from animal sources also have a relatively high content of sodium but, as the healthy diet pyramid indicates, we should all decrease our intake of animal products.

Milk, being an animal protein product, falls into this group and the recommended intake for an adult is 300 ml and, generally, this should not be exceeded.

High Sodium Items

- All canned, corned, and pickled meat or salted meat or fish. All processed meat e.g. Corned beef, salami, chicken loaf, ham, bacon, sausages, Frankfurt, and tinned fish unless labelled no added salt.
- All hard cheese, especially Parmesan or Romano. Highly salted breakfast cereals, commercial cakes, pastries, buns, cake mixes. Take care with commercial dry biscuits and sweet biscuits, which can contain significant amounts of sodium.
- All canned vegetables unless labelled no added salt. Pickles, sauerkraut, minted frozen peas.
- All takeaway foods.
- All canned and packet soups, prepared sauces or sauce mixes, gravy powders, stock cubes, meat extracts, yeast extracts, vegetable salts, celery salt, garlic salt, lemon pepper, monosodium glutamate, commercial mayonnaise or salad dressings, commercial sauces, soy sauce, olives, salted nuts, snack foods e.g., potato crisps, meat and fish pastes, ordinary peanut butter.
- Milk chocolate, caramels, Dutch liquorice, fizzy lollies.

Alcohol

Like sugar, alcohol gives a false stimulus to the system and is rapidly followed by sedation and depression of certain body functions. It depletes the levels of vitamins, most notably the B group, and C, and minerals, such as zinc, magnesium and potassium.

It is fashionable to imbibe alcohol and an increasing number of women are resorting to this practice although it has been found that the harmful effects of alcohol on women far exceeds those on men.

Eventually, alcohol takes a heavy toll on health, causing cirrhosis of the liver, gastric troubles, heart disease, muscle disorders, nervous system problems, sexual impotence, etc.

If natural fruit juices are kept warm for a few days and exposed to the air, the sugars in them will usually ferment to form alcohol.

Alcohol, to the chemist, is a general name; the alcohol we drink is called ethyl alcohol. Ordinary beers contain between 2½ and 4% of this alcohol by volume; special strong beers may have as much as 8%. Wines generally range between 8-12%, and fortified wines (e.g. sherries and aperitifs) contain added spirits, which bring the alcohol content up to about 20%.

Social drinking within limits is not harmful but it is the problem of alcoholism, which can be hazardous.

What is Alcoholism?

Alcoholic drinks provide a source of energy for the body but contain relatively few nutrients and vitamins. Those who drink them moderately, in company, are 'social drinkers'. Some social drinkers become heavy drinkers, and may develop, without necessarily recognizing it, into excessive drinkers. These are people whose drinking leads to social, economic or medical problems. Alcoholism is a self-inflicted condition but its effects are not confined to the individual drinkers. It breaks up marriages, alienates children and loses people their jobs. Physically the effects can be disastrous. It is thought that around 70% of chronic alcoholics suffer from fatty infiltration of the liver and about 10% from cirrhosis of the liver.

Nutritional Values of Alcohol

Alcohol contains traces of vitamins and minerals, but its nutritional contribution to the diet is negligible. Beer, for example, is a relatively poor source of carbohydrates compared with fruit juice. And wine contains small amounts of niacin, riboflavin, iron, calcium, and potassium, but richer sources of these nutrients are found in foods.

Because of its low nutritional content, alcohol is often described as providing 'empty' calories, but this doesn't mean they are few in number. Pure alcohol contains 7 calories per gram – fewer than fat but more than carbohydrates and protein. If you are trying to control your weight, consider that for the same 150 calories in a can of beer, you could eat a medium size baked potato, or 2 slices of whole grain bread.

Effects on Health

- Chronic heavy drinking is linked with an increased risk of cancer of the mouth, throat, oesophagus, liver, pancreas and rectum. The risk is heightened if a heavy drinker is also a smoker. Several studies have suggested that women who consume alcohol even moderately (as few as three drinks a week) have a higher risk of developing breast cancer than women who don't drink.

- Many alcoholics have peptic ulcers. A regular drinking causes chronic inflammation of the stomach, which in turn causes most alcoholics to lose interest in food. As a result of eating a small amount of convenience food, alcoholics often consume a diet low in vitamin content. They may nevertheless maintain a normal weight or increase in weight because alcohol substitutes for carbohydrates in the diet.
- Excessive alcohol may also weaken the heart muscle, causing the heart to enlarge and reducing the efficiency of the pumping action. Eating a balanced diet may protect a heavy
- Drinker from some of these effects, but not all. Another effect is the nerve damage described as polyneuritis- a tingling in the hands and feet, and cramps in the legs, are among the symptoms –which may affect a fifth of all alcoholics.
- Some of the neurological complications, such as the 'shakes' and delirium tremens (hallucinations), are 'withdrawal symptoms', and alcoholics who have reached this stage need hospital treatment under special care. Others –severe memory loss, for example – may be permanent.
- Chronic heavy drinking has serious impact on how the body absorbs, uses and stores food. Alcohol is metabolised by the liver, a process that takes precedence over other liver functions and interferes with that organ's effectiveness in processing nutrients. In a chronic heavy drinker, fat is stored in the liver instead of being metabolised efficiently. As a result, the liver grows larger and its ability to metabolise many vitamins and minerals is impaired. Damage to the pancreas, stomach, and gastrointestinal tract due to chronic heavy drinking may also hinder the absorption of nutrients.
- Vitamin and mineral deficiencies, particularly that of magnesium, calcium, phosphorus, zinc, pyridoxine, thiamine, riboflavin, niacin, folic acid and vitamins A, C and D, have been noted in alcoholics.

- Heavy drinking also leads to reduced dexterity. Alcohol is very rapidly absorbed and begins to act on the brain in about ten minutes. Co-ordination of hand and eye begins to fail, as does the ability to judge distance precisely and the brain function required to drive a motorcar or operate powered machinery safely.

Although these kinds of co-ordination fail and sometimes brain damage can be permanent, verbal skill usually remains unaffected. So do not regard your ability to talk coherently as proof of your ability to drive safely. Drinking is also an important cause of accidents and violence both at work and home.

However, these physical and mental effects are complications of alcohol misuse and generally arise only years after the sufferer's personal, social and professional life has been destroyed. Care should be taken so that one does not reach that stage.

Junk Food

Now that we know the foods that are damaging to our health, let us find out why everyone trashes the junk food. Fast food or junk food, as it is called, has all the elements of the damaging foods that are so hazardous to our health. It is also a misconception that only western food is junk food. In fact, *pakoras, bhelpuri, chaat, samosa* etc. also fall under the same category although the calories contained in them may not be as high as that in a hamburger or a pizza.

It is true that they are rich in the protein factors since many of them like hamburgers, rolls, hot dogs etc, contain a certain amount of fish, meat, chicken or bean component. They may even provide some vitamins but what they supply in excess are factors that can be harmful. What are these harmful factors?

One thing they provide in plenty is the calories. Whether it is the burger, the rolls, the pizza or the French fries, the number of calories they contain is enormous. Just one portion of the junk food item is enough to give calories required for the entire day. And if you take the help of some aerated soft drinks to gulp the fast food down, there are some more calories get added to the kitty.

The worst part is that most of the calories come from fat. Ingredients like cheese, butter, mayonnaise and the deep-frying of most of the other elements, add liberally to the fat content in the fast foods. The layer of cheese, mayonnaise, butter that goes into the pizza topping is bad news for the heart. And heaven help those of you, trying to reduce weight. The other factor against deep-frying is that the oil is generally recycled. Everyone knows that recycled oil is carcinogenic in nature so whether you are having '*chaat*', burger with cutlets or *samosa,* the cancer factor is very active.

What is common in noodles, pizza, samosa, cakes, burgers and hot dogs? Foxed? They all contain refined flour, which has no fibre, whatsoever. Refined flour has nothing to recommend it. It is a big zero, nutritionally with the additional ill effect of clogging up the intestines. So why settle for something that has nothing in it except a whole lot of calories?

Wait, there is still more danger in the fast food that you are gorging on. Most of the ingredients in the junk foods are canned, or bottled, the ketchup for instance or the mayonnaise or the sausage, ham and salami contain food additives, which are known hazards and carcinogenic elements. Additives such as emulsifiers, antioxidants, stabilisers, anti-caking agents, preservatives and taste enhancers contain chemicals that have been proven to cause diseases to human beings. Apart from these elements, short shelf life, inadequate quality check, unhealthy cooking conditions and handling, all add to the hazardous nature of the fast or junk food.

Let us just take a look at the two medium slices of pepperoni pizza you are consuming with great relish. The base is made of refined flour with food additives to make it rise. The calorie count is 640 kcal; apart from the calories, your pizza contains 36 gms of fat and 1898 mg of sodium. It also contains other food additives that have been added to cheese to preserve and emulsify it. Hidden factors of sodium are also present in the ketchup along with some more food chemicals.

Want to top it up with some fries and soft drinks? Add 200 calories for the fries alone and the whole gamut of food additives, as well as sugar in the soft drink. Oh! I forgot to take the caffeine into account.

Do you still want to take your family out to the nearest pizza place?

■ ■

Chapter 4

THE ANTI-AGEING FOOD PLAN

The Anti-Ageing food plan focuses on organically grown, unprocessed, chemical-free foods selected from the Four Food Groups consisting of grains, legumes, fruits, and vegetables.

This diet is not only naturally low in fat but also naturally high in desirable complex carbohydrates. In fact, approximately eighty percent of the calories you consume in a day should come from complex carbohydrates such as whole-grain breads, cereals, pastas, brown rice, potatoes, yams, and squash. The other twenty percent of calories should come from protein and fat, in equal portions.

Eating this way automatically eliminates the free radical burden imposed by a high-fat diet. It also sidesteps other known toxins, including pesticides, food additives, alcoholic beverages, and sugar. By following this diet plan, you can protect your immune and cardiovascular systems from damage, prevent diseases of degeneration, and slow the ageing process.

By adhering to the diet plan, you accomplish two goals. First, you boost your intake of disease-fighting essential nutrients, antioxidants, phytochemicals, and fibre—the substances that reinforce your body's healing powers, increase its resistance to disease, and extend life span. Second, you sidestep disease-causing substances like fats, sugar, white flour, pesticides, antibiotics, hormones, additives, and preservatives that undermine health and shorten life span.

Foods to Include

Before you begin the anti-ageing food plan, you have to make a commitment to stick with the diet that will substitute the meats, the dairy products, and the highly refined and processed fare with the following foods:

Grains – What you need is a diet, which is high in complex carbohydrates and low in protein and fat. So you'll be getting many of your daily calories from grains such as wheat, rye, oats (oatmeal and oat bran), millet, rice (brown, not white), and corn. For the most nutritional value, stick with organic, whole, minimally processed grains and grain products as much as possible.

Legumes – Legumes are seed- pods—beans, peas, lentils, and the like. Stock your pantry with all kinds: adzuki beans, anasazi beans, black beans, brown beans, chickpeas, green beans, green peas, kidney beans, lima beans, mung beans, navy beans, pinto beans, and, of course, soybeans and soy products (such as tofu, tempeh, and soy milk).

Fruits – You can't go wrong in this group, either—simply choose whatever is in season. Fresh fruits are preferable to frozen, since the freezing process can destroy some of the nutrients. As for juices, purchase organic products made from whole fruits or try making your own from organically grown whole fruits. Avoid juices made from concentrate as well as those with added sugar or with preservatives.

Vegetables – Vegetables are the most nutritious elements in an anti-ageing diet plan. They're also the best sources of protective phytochemicals. We are fortunate to have so many varieties of vegetables in our country. There is a whole range of green, yellow and red vegetables to choose from. No matter which ones you choose, you'll get bountiful amounts of vitamins, minerals, phytochemicals, and fibre. It is always a good idea to plan a menu, which includes vegetables of all colours because that is the easiest way of ensuring that most of the vitamins and other essentials are available to you.

Beets, broccoli, Brussels sprouts, cabbage, carrots, cauliflower, eggplant, garlic, green beans, kale, leeks, onions, peas, peppers (all kinds), potatoes (sweet and white), spinach, sprouts (all kinds), squash (all kinds), string beans, and tomatoes are especially recommended for their nutritional value. One extra beneficial factor could be added by buying organically grown vegetables.

Foods to Skip

An anti-ageing diet plan has no place for foods like red meat, poultry, milk, cheese, and eggs. Thousands of studies indict these foods for their role in the current epidemic of heart disease, cancer, and other degenerative conditions. For longevity, and youthful life, you will have to avoid all animal foods.

Similarly, refined carbohydrates such as white sugar, white flour, and processed foods are also a taboo for those following the anti-ageing diet. Refined carbohydrates have had their vitamins, minerals, and fibre stripped away, so they're of little nutritional value.

In contrast, complex carbohydrates like wheat, brown rice etc. are good because they retain their nutrients and they're converted to blood sugar more slowly. This prevents fluctuations in your blood sugar level, reduces fat storage, and supports weight loss and maintenance. As a bonus, when you eat a lot of complex carbohydrates, your diet automatically becomes low in fat and protein. In fact, because the foods have such good nutritional profiles, you can eat as much as you like.

Foods to be Avoided

Meats	Canned, salted or smoked meat, fish, bacon, cold cuts, chipped or corned beef, frankfurters, ham, sausage, frozen fish fillets, clams, lobsters, crabs, oysters, scallops, and shrimp.
Cereals	Quick cooking cereals, enriched cereals containing sodium compounds.
Breads and starches	Regular breads, hot breads and pastries prepared with baking soda or regular baking powder, cakes and mixes.
Vegetables	Frozen green peas, lima beans, and vegetable juice.
Fruits and juices	Crystallised or glazed fruit, dried or frozen fruit with sodium sulphite or sodium benzoate added and regular tomato juice.

Fats	Salted butter or margarine, bacon, olives, salted nuts, commercial mayonnaise, peanut better and cheese, French dressings etc.
Milk	Powdered, condensed, evaporated, buttermilk.
Beverages	Instant cocoa mixes and mineral water.
Sweets	Brown sugar, molasses, commercial syrups, candies, jams, and jellies containing sodium preservatives.
Desserts	Baking mixes, commercial ice-creams etc.
Miscellaneous	Mustard, pickles, chilli sauce, meat sauces, relishes, soy sauce, and monosodium glutamate.

Persons with severe cardiac conditions should avoid the following gas forming foods – broccoli, cauliflower, cabbage, Brussels sprouts, Cole slaw, green peppers, onions, corn, cucumbers, radishes, turnips, sweet potatoes, melon, raw apples and lima beans. Avoid the stimulating beverages like strong coffee, and strong tea also.

Supplements

What are the supplements that might help turn back the hands of time?

Vitamin E should be top on your list of supplements to consider. Not only are there hundreds of studies showing this vitamin lowers heart-disease risk, but recent evidence suggests it also might help protect your memory. The brain is exposed to a hefty dose each day of oxygen fragments called free radicals that damage the membranes and components of brain cells, possibly contributing to memory loss as we age. People who consume hefty doses of anti-free radicals or antioxidants also show the least memory loss and the best concentration as they age. Even animals fed on diets fortified with vitamin E learn faster and remember more. Limited evidence suggests that vitamin E also might slow the progression of Alzheimer's disease.

How Much Should You Take?

You can get some vitamin E from nuts, seeds, and oils, but not enough to prevent ageing. A safe supplemental dose is between 100IU and 400IU. Natural vitamin E is more potent than synthetic vitamin E.

Besides Vitamin E, What other Supplements are Worth Considering?

Calcium. I know you've heard it before, but people still need to be reminded to boost their calcium intakes to lower their risk for not only osteoporosis, but possibly colon cancer and hypertension, and pre-eclampsia in pregnancy.

If you don't drink at least three glasses of non-fat milk or cups of yoghurt, or drink calcium-fortified soymilk or orange juice, then you need to take a calcium supplement. Since most people get at least 600mg from their diets, you really only need to fill in the gaps by taking about 500mg from a supplement.

Which Ones are the Best?

Either calcium carbonate or calcium citrate supplies the most calcium per pill. You also need vitamin D, so make sure your multi-vitamin contains 200IU to 400IU of this vitamin, which is essential for calcium absorption and getting the calcium into bones.

Fish Oils

For millions of years, our ancestors ate diets rich in a type of fat called omega-3 fatty acids, the fats once found in wild game and now found primarily in fish oils. Estimates are that our ancestors consume an average of up to 10 grams a day, while today we consume less than one gram daily. While saturated fats in meat and dairy are storage-type fats, fish oils are structural fats that are important components of cell membranes and hormone-like compounds in the body that possibly protect against a host of ills, from heart disease and cancer to even memory loss and depression. Even babies need these fats to ensure normal brain and vision development. Although an optimal daily dose has not been identified, general consensus is at least two to three servings of fatty fish per week (salmon, mackerel, herring). Also, heart attack risk might decrease by 50 percent when people consume daily at least 200 mg of the omega-3 fatty acids in supplements or in foods.

Anti-Ageing Foods

Many of what are considered signs of ageing—wrinkled skin, a fading memory, diminished physical capacity and an increased susceptibility to infection—are actually little more than deficiencies of critical chemicals called antioxidants. You don't have to sit by and watch your body disintegrate. Instead, you can eat the following 10 foods to help hang on to and replenish your biomechanical vitality. Just about any fruit or vegetable will make contributions to your quest for youth; here are ten important ones, you shouldn't ignore.

1. ***Avocado:*** True, avocado is high in fat, much of it is "good" fat, the mono-unsaturated type, which resists oxidation. Avocado is high in glutathione, an antioxidant which helps neutralize fat in other foods. Research also suggests that eating avocado lowers and improves cholesterol better than a low-fat diet does.
2. ***Berries:*** Blueberries have more antioxidants called anthocyanins than any other food—in fact, 3 times more than the second-richest sources, red wine and green tea. Both blueberries and cranberries help ward off urinary tract infections. And a study showed that older people who ate strawberries had the lowest rates of all kinds of cancer.
3. ***Broccoli:*** The green stuff provides an awesome array of antioxidants. Scientists at John Hopkins Institute discovered a particularly strong one called sulforaphane. Served to animals, the broccoli chemical stoked the activity of detoxification enzymes that slashed cancer rates by two-thirds. Broccoli is packed with vitamin C, beta-carotene, indole, glutathione and lutein, and is also a rich source of the trace metal chromium, which is a life extender and protects against the ravages of out-of-control insulin and blood sugar.
4. ***Cabbage:*** People who ate cabbage once a week compared with once a month had only 66 percent of the risk of colon cancer, one study found. Cabbage also seems to deter stomach cancer. Savoy cabbage (the crinkly type) is the strongest one; you can eat it raw or lightly cooked, for the best effect.
5. ***Carrots:*** Carrots are legendary in fighting off ageing diseases. In a recent study, men eating a couple of carrots a day lowered blood cholesterol by 10 percent. Many studies pinpoint beta-carotene, carrots' main antioxidant asset, as a powerhouse against ageing and disease. People with low levels of beta-carotene in their blood are more apt to have heart attacks, strokes and various cancers.

6. ***Citrus fruit:*** The National Cancer Institute has called the orange the "complete package of every class of natural anticancer inhibitor known, including carotenoids, terpenes, flavenoids and vitamin C." Grapefruit, too, has a unique type of fibre that reduces cholesterol dramatically and may reverse the ageing disease atherosclerosis.
7. ***Grapes:*** Grapes contain 20 known antioxidants that work together to fend off oxygen free-radical attacks that promote disease and ageing, according to researchers at the University of California. The antioxidants are in the skin and the seeds, and the more colourful the skin, the greater the antioxidant punch.
8. ***Onions:*** They might give you bad breath, but they help prevent cancer, thin your blood (discouraging clots) and raise the good type (HDL) of cholesterol. Red and yellow onions (sorry, not the white ones) are the richest of all foods in quercetin, a celebrated antioxidant that inactivates cancer-causing agents, inhibits enzymes that spur cancer growth and has anti-inflammatory, antibacterial, anti-fungal and antiviral activity.
9. ***Spinach:*** Heavy in lutein, an anti-ageing agent which rivals beta-carotene for effectiveness, spinach also has beta-carotene plus a good dose of folic acid, a brain and artery protector.
10. ***Tomatoes:*** These are the richest source of lycopene, which new research suggests helps to preserve mental and physical functioning among the elderly. High levels of lycopene also reduce your risk of pancreatic cancer.

Do you want to Remain Young Forever?

Who doesn't? Here are some sure shot tips to keep you looking at least ten years younger than your age. A word of caution – don't expect miracles or overnight results, patience and discipline in following these rules will get you to reach the ultimate goal.

- Drink a glass of vegetable juice every day. Raw vegetable juice is full of both known and unknown antioxidants, which in turn help in reducing the free radical activity.
- Eat at least 5 servings of fruits and vegetables every day. The goodness of fruits and vegetables can never be undermined.

- Consume less oil. Excessive fat intake increases free radical activity. The excess fat that we consume in the form of oily snacks gets oxidised and rancid thereby producing a burst of free radical activity in the body. These free radicals are in excess of what the body can normally diffuse and cause ageing. Recycling the used oil is another harmful habit practised by most homemakers. It is a dangerous practise, to say the least.
- There are endless brands of tea in the market but making a choice for a better one can work wonders. Have you ever wondered how do the Japanese retain their youthful looks? Well, the answer is quite simple—they drink green tea and eat a lot of fish. If you want similar benefits, switch to green tea as it has lot of antioxidants.
- Avoid sugar and refined flour for the same reason.
- Stop smoking. Smoking can age people by ten years apart from playing havoc with their health. It ages the skin and brings on the wrinkles around the mouth and eyes.
- Eat up to ¾ of your capacity. This helps your digestive machinery to work better.

Include at least 2 calcium rich foods every day. It could be a bowl of low fat curd and some soya bean or bowl of rajma, chowli or channa. Curd helps to increase the friendly bacteria in your gastro intestine tract and also looks after your bone health. Soya bean, apart from helping you to maintain healthy bones, has innumerable health benefits.

- Exercise or take a brisk walk for 30-40 minutes regularly for at least 6 days a week.
- Stay involved with family and friends. Being loved and a sense of belonging work as shock absorbers and help rev up immunity.
- Maintain a positive outlook.
- Do what really makes you happy. Apart from this, doing meaningful work with honesty and living one's life in a conscientious, responsible way all contributes to inner peace and longevity.

Heart friendly Foods

Eat more Omega-3 Fatty Acids

Eat more fish as it contains omega-3 fatty acids, which is heart-friendly and can actually lengthen the span of your life. Research indicates that the Eskimos and Japanese who eat fish regularly have lower rates of heart disease. Fish oils are known to contain antioxidants that block the oxidation of fat and thereby free radical formation. They also unclog the arteries and help increasing the HDL (good) cholesterol. But deep-frying the fish counteracts its anti-ageing properties. So either steam or poach the fish or prepare a fish curry. Choose sardine, mackerel and tuna.

Vegetarians can get the benefit of omega-3 fatty acids in certain plant foods namely wheat germ oil, walnut oil, almond oil, flaxseed oil and soybean oil.

Vitamin E for Vitality

Vitamin E, by virtue of its antioxidant property, hinders oxidation of bad cholesterol, prevents it from entering the arterial wall and reduces the incidence of heart attack.

The Goodness of Garlic

Studies have shown that eating raw garlic can reduce harmful blood fats. Garlic also combats acidity and gas formation when taken along with warm water on an empty stomach in the morning. The garlic that has only one clove has these medicinal properties.

Brain Foods

The brain is the largest consumer of the energy that our body produces. To process information efficiently, to access important data, to store necessary information, it needs oxygen, glucose and other nutrients. Lack of these leads to short-term memory loss and mental fatigue.

Symptoms of sluggishness, lethargy, dizziness and even fainting can occur if we don't feed the brain. The free radicals generated by the body could lead to erosion in the functioning of the brain.

Free radicals and antioxidants are two words that we are increasingly hearing in context of health and ageing. Few of us really understand these terms. Let us try to get a clearer picture about antioxidants and free radicals.

A freshly cut apple will turn brown in a matter of minutes. Iron, when exposed to water and air, starts to rust. These chemical changes are the result of oxidation, the process by which a compound reacts with oxygen. Oxidation in the body creates free radicals in the fats, tissues, and bloodstream.

Antioxidants are compounds that neutralize free radicals by giving them the necessary electron they crave. Antioxidants can be vitamins, minerals, hormones, or enzymes. Although a certain amount is manufactured in the body as enzymes or hormones, most of our antioxidants come from fruits and vegetables. Here are some anti-oxidants which are required by our body.

Vitamin C

Probably the most well known antioxidant, vitamin C helps minimize free radical damage to the neurological system. It also protects other antioxidants in the body, such as vitamin E. In addition to neutralizing free radicals, vitamin C detoxifies the body, reduces high blood pressure, lowers cholesterol, and fights cancer.

It has the beneficial effect on glutathione levels and helps prevent free radical damage to the brain cells.

Vitamin A and Beta-carotene

Both vitamin A and beta-carotene are powerful free-radical scavengers that help the skin, mucous membranes, circulatory system, and cholesterol levels. In particular, beta-carotene is very effective in neutralizing the singlet oxygen-free radical.

More than 600 different types of carotene have been identified from fruits and vegetables, only a few of which have been studied. Preliminary research indicates that alpha-carotene is up to 100 times more powerful as an antioxidant than beta-carotene. Others include lutein, gamma-carotene, zeaxanthin, and lycopene, a known cancer fighter that occurs in high concentrations in tomato products.

Vitamin E

This antioxidant prevents the oxidation of lipids (fats) in cell membranes, which strengthens the outer cell layers against free radical attack. Vitamin E works best in the presence of selenium, another antioxidant, and helps protect vitamin A. Vitamin E stimulates the immune system, improves the circulatory system and oxygen absorption, fights cancer, and has a role in preventing cataracts.

Vitamin E helps to protect the brain against oxidative stress. An intake of about 400 mg every day can be very helpful.

Lycopene

There is no question today that antioxidants are a significant part of the important nutrients we need today to support our health. One of the more newly understood of these antioxidants is lycopene. This much-hailed phytonutrient is found in tomatoes. It is actually the substance that gives tomatoes their red colour and, like beta-carotene, is a member of the carotene family.

Selenium

Selenium is in news. Every health magazine and newspaper has been going ga-ga about its values. It has been found to be beneficial in the fight against free radicals, which contribute to premature ageing, among other things. Selenium is found in the highest concentrations in seafoods, grains, muscle meats, and Brazil nuts. A multi-vitamin that contains between 70-100 mcg is recommended, but an additional supplement is not necessary. It has also recently shown that selenium can help prevent cancer.

Zinc

Just like it protects your car from rust, zinc has antioxidant properties that protect the body. Zinc is required to maintain effective levels of vitamins E and A. It is also a key ingredient in the very important antioxidant enzyme called superoxide dismutase (SOD).

Other Plant Sources

Several popular supplements like bilberry, brahmi, ginkgo biloba, Siberian ginseng and garlic are very strong antioxidants. Bilberry helps eliminate free radicals from capillary walls and red blood cells; it is also known to improve arthritis. Its ability to improve vision was first observed during World War II when it was discovered that British pilots, who ate bilberry jam, had excellent twilight vision.

Indian herb Brahmi contains substances called bacosides, which are responsible for improving memory and memory-related functions by enhancing the efficiency of nerve impulse transmission. Bacosides work by repairing damage to worn-out neurons.

Ginkgo biloba and Siberian Ginseng are famous for improving memory, partly because they contains antioxidants that scavenge free radicals and boost the effectiveness of vitamin C. They are also used to improve circulation, heart conditions, and neurological disorders such as Alzheimer's disease.

Garlic contains high amounts of antioxidants, vitamin A, vitamin C, carotene, and selenium and boosts the levels of antioxidant enzymes in the bloodstream. Consuming a couple of cloves of garlic may keep your friends away but they definitely help to protect the neurons from damage.

Green tea also contains a variety of antioxidants, including catechin, and is known to lower cholesterol levels and reduce blood clotting. Is it a wonder that the Japanese, who consume so much of green tea, are so brainy?

■■

Section Three YOUTHFUL LIFESTYLE

Modern lifestyle is the main culprit in causing an unfit body. The wrong kind of food, lack of exercise, the excessive stress factor and the neglect of the body, all add up to drive the final nail on the coffin of health.

In most homes, Sundays are a day for special meals and in our country a special meal is almost always something, which has a lot of oil and spices. Apart from the Sundays, there is always a celebration. The Indian calendar is full of festivities and each festival is observed by eating special food and sweets. Other than the festivals there are the birthdays, anniversaries, religious and social functions, parties etc. which provide people with an excuse to indulge in a food-orgy.

Lifestyle is not just about your food habits. It has to do with every aspect of your life, your activities at work and leisure, your intellectual development and your spiritual pursuits. A fast paced life, which brings about excessive stress, has also brought with it the ills of stress related diseases. Instead of simplifying the life and learning the art of living, we are rushing towards a state of ultimate disaster.

Investments in wealth are of no use if your health is not going to stand in good stead. Of what use are the lacs of rupees if we are not able to enjoy a fruitful and healthy life. A far wiser option is to invest in health. The moment one is able to understand this fact; he is on the right path. Working long hours, snatching hurried meals, consuming all kinds of stimulants and alcohol or smoking packs of cigarette to combat stress, disturbed sleep, pumping adrenaline, all this can but add to the woes of our systems. Balance and control is the key to a healthy living.

Chapter 1

HEALTH AND LIFESTYLE

The concept of preventive health is one that the great majority of people tend to ignore. Most of us are simply not tuned to the idea of protecting ourselves against possible illness. We tend to think of health as the absence of disease and when we become unwell we blame our illness on external factors, such as germs, extremes of weather, or crowded places. We dissociate our health from the general pattern of our lifestyles and, once recovered from an illness, we carry on regardless, continuing to live as we have always done. Yet, with a little thought and forward planning, most of us could protect ourselves from a great number of unnecessary ailments. And, what is more, we could positively enhance our health and vitality.

The most obvious way of enhancing our well being is by paying attention to our diet, but sufficient exercise and proper breathing and relaxation techniques are equally important. A responsible attitude to personal and sexual hygiene, and to the management of our home environment, is also essential – not only for our own health, but for the well-being of our families, too.

Changing Your Lifestyle

Changing lifestyle does not mean changing your entire personality. What it involves is an awareness of health in all areas of your life. Basic health diet and the fitness programmes should allow for gradual change. Radical, sudden changes would undoubtedly be stressful – and probably wouldn't last.

Even small steps towards a healthier lifestyle can prove immensely rewarding. When you start a new exercise programme, for instance, you may well find that your appetite is more easily regulated, and that you have less desire to smoke or drink (if these are problems for you). Regularly practising a relaxation technique, too, though it may take only a few minutes each day, will reduce the need for stimulants, encourage better sleep and, by releasing the energy locked up in stress, increase your vitality.

Preventive Health Care

A good diet, a balance of activity and rest, and time to devote to your mental and emotional well-being – all these elements amount to a preventive health care strategy. It is not just at the most serious diseases that preventive health care is aimed. Taking the responsibility for your own welfare includes the simplest of daily activities, such as brushing your teeth to prevent tooth decay or washing your hands before preparing food. On a calendar basis, it means regular health check ups – having your blood pressure tested at intervals and so on.

Diet

In the past decade, greater wealth has led to increased consumption of processed, high sugar and high fat foods, foods that were once regarded as luxuries. There has been a correspondingly sharp decline in the consumption of plain nutritious staples. The general quality has altered too, with modernisation in the food industry involving chemical additives and refining techniques, which have 'denatured' much of the food items.

Fortunately, the nutritional component in enhancing health and preventing, even curing illness is now widely recognised. It is well known that a poor diet can exacerbate stress, cause nervous disorders, and affect mental as well as physical development. There is also increasing concern about food allergies, and about the possibility of the potentially toxic cocktail of food additives reacting in the body.

Obesity, too, is a matter of widespread anxiety. It is one of the most serious risk factors in many types of illness and although there is a genetic element, it is largely a result of poor dietary habits. One of the marks of having "made it" in our society is the ability to eat out as frequently as possible and to consume all kinds of trash food. Obesity has arisen from inappropriate lifestyle selection habits, of which a part is inappropriate nutritional selection habits. Some cheeseburger with fries and a large soft drink alone can constitute upward of 1500 calories and this is what is the favoured food when one wants to spend an evening out with the friends. Fast food joints are promoting their ware by offering giant size soft drinks or complementary soft drinks to draw the crowds of eager youngsters. Is this the kind of eating habit one would like to promote in our youngsters?

One classic example of today's philosophy is the phrase –'living life king size'. This suggests that we have only one time around and we had better do it up right, because there may be no tomorrow. We gorge ourselves with food that is fit to be trashed, party all night, work all day, stimulate our senses with stimulants like coffee, tea or alcohol, load our systems with carbonated drinks, stress ourselves beyond the healthy limits and feel good about it. Not for a minute do we pause to think of the consequences. "This is living, man! And you only live once", we tell ourselves. We limp slowly off into the sunset after some 20 years of significant debilitation.

Is this what living is all about? Is this the life you visualise for yourself? At this minute you may not even realise what I am talking about but when you are fifty and the body starts rebelling against the ill-treatment you have heaped on it, you will realise the folly of having lived the king-size life.

With the influence of the globalisation and westernisation, more and more Indians are falling prey to unhealthy food habits. Fast foods like pizza, hamburgers, colas and French fries have replaced the healthy Indian foods like idli, chapatti and upma. Sandwiches have replaced the normal *chapati-sabzi* in the lunch boxes of most adults as well as children. Breads, not necessarily brown bread, have become popular due to lack of time in working women's kitchens. All this is bound to have an unhealthy effect on the present and future generations.

Challenges of Modern Lifestyle

The problems faced by people today, have become much more complex than before. Society has become more complicated.

Somehow, the concept of economic "success" has replaced the traditional values of human bonding, of communication with nature, of a deep knowledge of life, and of what is important in sustaining life and cultivating wisdom. Economic success has replaced what brings true happiness, and it has done so at the inconceivable expense of the land and the environment that supports life. Technological "success" has been at the unfathomable expense of the people, of whole cultures, and ways of life born out of the wisdom of the ages, which, for centuries, supported mankind, high cultural expression, and supreme spiritual life, especially among the people of Asian countries.

Gone is the communion of people with each other, with the animals, the land, plants, trees, mountains, water, and spirits. Gone is the knowledge of invisible things, the greater part of us. How small we have made ourselves, when we focus only on the seen, the tangible. We see only what is outside, not what is within. We have clearly forgotten to respect and revere nature.

Meanwhile, the very chemicals that are creating cancer, birth defects, and deaths, continue to be used on the foods, which the public eats.

The macrobiotic way of natural and organic agriculture avoids the problem altogether. As more people support organic agriculture, the chemical agricultural industry will dry up and wither away. Organic farming has sufficiently proven its validity and ability to sustain us, in the delicious and nutritional quality of the food, freedom from pests, and economic stability.

We need not lose sight of the greater, higher path of a natural, macrobiotic, way of life. The more we study the traditional teachings and ways of life of traditional cultures worldwide, the deeper our understanding of macrobiotics becomes. Such study cultivates a multidimensional understanding of life, as perceived and practiced by indigenous peoples everywhere.

Therefore, people with no life-threatening illness can protect their health by gradually, and comfortably, transitioning into a regimen of whole grains and vegetables, diminishing red meat and dairy, occasionally using a little fowl, and finally substituting all animal foods with fish. Fish can be enjoyed once or twice a week, with grains and vegetables, and a small salad, with some fresh or cooked fruits for dessert. This pattern can be followed for several months, or years, as one prefers.

These days, illnesses are more complex and take more time to heal, due to the introduction of complex chemical pollutants and contaminants, as well as synthetic drugs and medicines, into the environment, our food supplies, and our bodies. Before the extent of all this contamination, manipulation, and industrialization of our foods and the environment took place, the body could heal faster. Now it takes longer for some problems to reverse. Still, right food is the best medicine.

Secondary treatments may be helpful from time to time, such as herbs, massage, acupuncture, homeopathy, or, sometimes, some form of medical intervention, but nothing is as basic, fundamental, and transformative as food. Ideally, if food is correct nothing else is necessary.

We live in a time of traumatic transitions. Many people need some form of psycho-spiritual counselling, or way of life guidance, to enable them to pursue a stable macrobiotic practice. We bring many unresolved problems, conflicts, and addictions into our macrobiotic practice without knowing how to handle them. They do not all dissolve automatically just because we start eating brown rice. Appropriate dietary adjustment is essential and effective, but discharge (catharsis) and purification at the heart and soul level are also important.

Art of Living

We have forgotton the art of living. We live on the judgments made using the sense organs that distinguish colour, shape, distance, sound, smell, taste, and touch. This stage of nerve function is instantaneous and spontaneous and does not require the consciousness of higher brain function. At this stage, there is no time for thinking; reactions are like reflexes, they operate instantly. Therefore, this stage of thinking exists in even the simplest creatures such as insects, fish, and snails. In humans, these sensorial reflections are slower and less sharp than those of simpler creatures since humans with their higher brain functions are always thinking and assersing things.

However, some humans do not use their higher brain functions to think, but use them only for sensorial reflection. They behave with emotion, but not with reason. Their goals in life focus on nice clothes, better cars, better houses, tasty foods, better sex, and other conveniences and comforts.

Often, at the end of these pleasures are financial difficulties, sicknesses, arguments, anger, resentment, and jealousy. Since those people live according to reflex senses, they cannot overcome or change difficulties in their life. In order to change difficulties to happiness, we need endurance, which requires more than the sensorial level or stage of consciousness.

One who lives according to the senses does not use the higher brain functions, which require endurance. Therefore, when they encounter difficulties, they are desperate, disappointed, and unhappy. So, the first condition to be able to live a happy life is endurance.

Someone who has no endurance cannot overcome difficulties. To overcome difficulties one has to try hard, especially after failing a few times, and never give up, to be able to transform unhappiness to happiness.

If you want to be happy, don't try to be perfect or always first. This desire, taken to an extreme, can create enormous stress in your life and can lead to arrogance. This stress and arrogance can create an emotional quick-sand that will rob you of good quality energy and will sap your endurance.

Do only what you really want to do. Quit your job if you don't like it and find something else to do. Don't stay in an unhappy place. However, those who have developed a high sense of endurance always manage to rise up above the situations and are always in control. Life goals pursued for mundane reasons like money, power or status are likely to make you unhappy.

Evaluating Your Lifestyle

By the time you have come to this part of the book you must have realised the impact that nutrition and life-style can have on your health, and you have also been sensitised to some of the variables which you can adjust to frame a more healthy lifestyle.

The first thing that matters is the realisation that the lifestyle you are following is not really the best. Once you have realised that, you have to follow it up with a conviction that you have to do something about it, Now the question is – where do I begin and how do I do it?

Once we have convinced ourselves that we are ultimately responsible for our own state of health, we are ready to explore our own lifestyle. Before that, one must know that a change in lifestyle alone does not guarantee that you will never be ill. All it guarantees is that you will be far healthier than you presently are. To assess you lifestyle, make a checklist, which includes the following areas:

1. Diet
2. Activity
3. Leisure
4. The work-place environment
5. Level of intellectual stimulation

1. Dietary Evaluation

The first thing that you need to do is to record all the foods that you eat for a weeklong period. Make this period a time in which you are not eating irregularly or consuming food that is not your normal kind. Look for the frequency of various kinds of foods that are high in sugar content or high in fat. Look for how often you eat out, what kinds of beverage you consume. Are they sugar-rich, alcoholic, low in calcium, low in other vitamins or minerals? Look at foods that have high residue in your diet, such as the fibre-rich whole grains and vegetables.

How do you Prepare and Consume Those Foods?

- Are they parboiled or deep-fried?
- Do you consume freshly prepared food or do you heat and reheat it?
- Do you generally consume a certain kind of vegetables, such as green leafy vegetable with their inherent B vitamins, magnesium and vitamin C content?
- Do you look for milk and milk products and for foods that are reasonably low in fat and high in complex carbohydrates.

- How frequent is your consumption of non-vegetarian food?
- Do you snack more while watching the television or entertaining friends?
- What kind of snacks do you prefer?

All these questions can be easily answered by inspecting your dietary record. Be sure, however, to include everything you consume, snacks and beverages, also.

What is your emotional investment in eating?

- Do you eat excessively when you are bored or depressed?
- Do you eat foods that you know are 'bad' for you?
- Do you prefer eating alone?
- Do you sneak or hid food?
- Do you have feelings of being rushed or a sense of urgency, when you are eating?
- Do you have feeling of being caught in the midst of a struggle with your diet in order to maintain weight?
- Do you have uncontrollable hunger urges?
- Do you tend to stuff yourself whenever food is put in front of you?

All the above questions reflect your emotional involvement in the process of eating. Analyse them well. If your answer to most of them is 'yes', it is time for you to evaluate your psychological investment in eating.

2. Activity Record

Keeping an activity record of atleast a week can be quite interesting. Keep track of how you spend your time for those seven days.

- How much time do you sleep?
- How much time do you spend in sedentary activities?
- How much time do you spend in physical activities like walking, jogging etc?
- How much of your time is spent in leisure activities and what are they?
- I bet most of us do not even know what we pack into our 24 hours.

Maintaining the record could be an eye-opener. Many times this kind of time motion study can point up very important facts or excess of various types of activities, which can stimulate weight gain, stress, anxiety or overeating.

The activity record is an extremely important way of analysing how you programme your daily activities and how many calories of energy you expend in activity. It is also important to record on this activity record the times that you eat, to see if there is any association between snacking and certain activities. If, in fact, you regularly consume biscuits, coffee or soft drinks after you have been sitting at your desk for about 3 hours, then this establishes a behaviour pattern, which may contribute to over consumption. You can easily break the pattern by structuring your time so that you take a walk around or engage in another activity after an hour of sitting at the desk.

We all have woven into our lifestyles certain kinds of eating and activity habit that relate to our past experiences. These can generally be understood only if they are written down and examined later.

3. Leisure Log

As you are completing the diet survey and activity records, you should also keep a leisure log. A leisure log is a record of how you have allocated your leisure time.

- Do you spend your leisure time in front of the television in a state of intellectual stupor, or is it spent in developing some new skill or refining a talent?
- Does you leisure time lead you to feelings of contribution and of relaxation?
- Do you feel refreshed and relaxed and ready to go after your leisure time activities or do they make you nervous and agitated?

A good example for some individuals is their golf game. Golf is ostensibly a leisure-time activity; however, the perfectionism that is brought to the game can by the 18th hole make people so anxious that their blood pressure is increased. This is not the kind of leisure that leads to stress reduction and maintenance of a good mind-body relationship.

A leisure log which denotes the way that you felt about a particular leisure time activity should allow you to explore why you partition your time in a certain way. An activity, which is contributing in some manner to your high-tension, distressful lifestyle, is not a very healthy one. If the leisure time activity really gives you a break from your normal, hectic life would be the one you need to pursue.

4. Workplace Environment

Spend two or three days analysing your work place environment. Examine the lighting that you work under, look at the quality of air that you breathe, look at the conditions of stress and potential distress. Remember light and air are nutrients that feed the body as surely as does food. Take some pulse reading at different time of the day, you should have a resting pulse of less than 80 beats per minute. If you are nervous your pulse rises in response.

- Count the number of coffee cups you consume at work. Are you consuming more than 3-4 cups and at what time?
- Look at your pattern of telephone usage. Do you get mad when you hear the phone ringing, does it interrupt you often?
- Do you feel bored?
- Is repetition too much a part of your daily workplace lifestyle?
- Do you spend long hours sitting either in an automobile or at a desk without the opportunity to move around?
- Is the environment noisy, dusty, polluted or depressing?

An in-depth analysis of your work place environment plays a significant role in determining the relationship you have with your own body and ultimately your health. You spend approximately two third of your day working or sleeping. Many of us accept whatever the work place environment doles out to us in terms of activities as given in our lives. We can adjust the kind of working place environment in which we find ourselves, but only if we recognise those things that are supporting our health and those that are really eroding our relationship with our bodies. Often, the adjustment comes at a very high price, that of our health.

5. Intellectual Stimulation

Just as food provides nutrition for the body, intellectual stimulation provides it to the mind. There is no way that we can operate effectively as human beings in a vacuum. We must set goals, which allow our minds to be enriched as well as our bodies. Without the stimulation our minds will wither and die. Setting new goals for intellectual stimulation and occasionally re-evaluating whether or not we are meeting them is extremely important.

We should have a certain commitment to music, sports, arts, crafts, language skill or literature that allow us to move into new intellectual areas and keep expanding? The most important single asset that we have, as an organism differentiated from the rest of the animal kingdom, is our brain. The brain is an extremely hungry organ that requires tremendous amount of energy to keep it nourished, yet it can pay back dividends if we are willing to use it effectively.

In putting together a healthy lifestyle, one must seek out sources, which continue to challenge new domains of the brain and capitalise on that unique gift that we were given as a species.

Only if we continue to get intellectual stimulation will we reach a state of self-actualisation that will finally get us in a state of joyful existence. The feeling that we are able to return something to the society and make a contribution to the world at large can lead us to the self-actualisation levels.

Towards a Healthier Lifestyle

Now that you have made a proper evaluation of your existing lifestyle, it is time to move towards a healthier one. By now you have realised where your strengths and deficiencies lie and it is time to make the changes and the positive reinforcements which encourage you to continue the change.

Any change that you make in your lifestyle which is designed to better your health will lead you closer to making many other changes. If you start eating better, it will not be too long until you start wanting to exercise or vice versa. The philosophical change that comes from making a commitment to your own health is the most important facet of the programme. The first corner you must turn, which is the largest corner, is to commit yourself to your own responsibility. Then you must design your environment to support the allocation of time to activities which you know are in your best interest and to minimise the time spent on activities which are well recognised as undermining your health. Your body knows how to eat right and live in a healthful way if you would only get out of its way.

When you know where the problem lies, it becomes so much easier to handle it. I bet you are in for a few shocks yourself when you read and evaluate your logs. You must never have really known what kind of food you are consuming, what are your daily activities like and how much time you spend doing things you like, in your spare time. It is like a whole new world has opened up before your eyes and you know exactly what you must do.

You do not need to become a nutrition nut and suddenly switch to lentils, tofu and soya as your main source of calories. Prudent dietary selection when you shop for food items can make a tremendous difference in the quality of nutrition. Try to use fundamental starting material as much as possible, such as whole grains, vegetables, legumes, and brown rice. Similarly, when you find that your activity log shows hardly any activity, you could start by introducing some nice calorie-burning activities. Or for that matter, if the leisure log indicates a complete vacuum in terms of hobbies, maybe its time to pick a challenging and satisfying one. Maybe you have some secret talents, which need to be nurtured, but you never found time or inclination to do so. Now is the time to do it.

Nothing will happen overnight, remember you have taken some 30-40 years to develop these habits. Changing them will come with time. But a slow commitment to a change in philosophy will help everyone to turn the corner and become friends again with their own bodies, working jointly toward optimising health and minimising the need for crisis medical intervention.

■■

Chapter 2

THE MACROBIOTIC LIFESTYLE

The term "macrobiotic" describes a holistic lifestyle, which seeks to empower people to take control of their lives and to educate them to make healthy lifestyle choices and decisions. It empowers individuals to establish awareness, health, and harmony in their lives, personal relationships, communities, and environment.

Macrobiotics is a holistic philosophy that aims to achieve balance and peace in people's lives through awareness and common sense living. Common sense living includes getting enough rest, eating the way nature intended, being kind and respectful towards one and others, and respecting the environment.

Macrobiotics is now popularly known for and has been well publicised for its success in curing disease, most notably cancer. While a very strict version of the macrobiotic diet can eliminate many cancers, most macrobiotic practitioners recommend a more varied diet based on whole grains, vegetables, beans, and other organic natural foods. By eating the way nature intended, you not only support the ecosystem, but also enhance your own health. To test this yourself, read our seasonal heath tip for easy ways you can transition to natural foods and feel stronger and healthier in the process!

Macrobiotics is based on the Chinese philosophy of *Yin* and *Yang,* which are two qualities that balance one; another, and which exist in every natural object and cycle. Yin (pronounced 'yeen') is the flexible, fluid and cool side of nature, while yang (pronounced 'yahn') elements in everything, including people, and macrobiotics is a philosophy aimed at balancing them to promote good health.

Yin qualities are peacefulness, calm, creativity, sociability and a relaxed attitude and behaviour. Yang qualities include activity, alertness, energy and precision. Most people have a mix of both these qualities. However, when one becomes stronger than the other, a state of imbalance can occur, which can result in illness. Too much yin can lead to depression, fatigue and sleeping problems; too much yang can cause tension, irritability, hyperactivity and insomnia.

A macrobiotic therapist would attempt to right that balance by suggesting an increased intake of yin foods for someone suffering from too much yang, and the opposite for someone with too much yin.

Achieving personal health and balance is the first step in realising harmony in all other relationships!

Macrobiotics - A Brief History

The Macrobiotic way is a school of thought and action, based upon the use of natural materials in our fabrics, our homes and our food. Even many naturally occurring ingredients can be hazardous to our health (e.g. hemlock, opium, sodium, lead); therefore, to determine the correct applications for natural materials, they are classified in accordance with the "Unique Principle".

The Unique Principle was introduced to the Western world by George Ohsawa (Yukikazu Sakurazawa), a Japanese businessman, teacher and writer. As a teenager, Ohsawa was diagnosed with tuberculosis and was deemed to have little chance of surviving. However, by following the teaching of Sagen Ishizuka, a natural healer who was famous in Japan near the beginning of the 20th century, Ohsawa was able to heal himself.

He travelled from Japan to Europe in 1929 and, soon thereafter, began teaching the Unique Principle.

The "Principle" itself, employs the ancient oriental practice of Yin and Yang theory, to determine the quality of the materials in our universe. Though all aspects of the environment are important in the macrobiotic way of thinking, there is a special emphasis on food. This is because the food we eat becomes our bodies. Therefore, special attention is paid to the quality of that portion of the environment, which we consume. All things, including food, can be classified into a “more yin” or a “more yang” category. Generally speaking, yin foods tend to be more sugary, watery, cold and tropical in origin. Yang foods tend to be more meaty, dry, cooked and polar in nature.

Very yang foods like mammal meat, poultry, table salt, ginseng as well as very yin foods like sugar, euphoric drugs, strong alcoholic beverages are generally avoided. These foods are often called Extreme Food. Balanced foods which are not so extreme compose the standard macrobiotic diet. Cereal grains, reside at the balance between yin and yang. Therefore, whole grains and their derivatives (pasta, bread, hominy) are considered the mainstay of the diet. All ancient civilisations had used a grain-based element as the main diet.

Along with whole grain, the diet is comprised of bean and bean products, a wide variety of vegetables, kelp and other sea vegetables, many excellent soups and condiments, nuts and occasional fish and fruit. Macrobiotic people pay close attention to their personal condition and they adjust the yin and yang quality of their diets, as required to maintain a healthy life and happiness. In addition to classification by type, the quality of the food is also considered. Vegetables should be organically grown.

Fish and sea vegetables should be harvested from deep, clean water or from coastal areas located far from city and industrial pollution. Also, genetically engineered foods, even grains and beans, are to be avoided. Organic food grown from traditional, open-pollinated seed is best. To some individuals, this entire process may sound unlikely or farfetched. In that case, it would be important to know that the Macrobiotic diet has healed thousands of individuals; some, from very life threatening illnesses, such as cancer and heart disease and has even enabled diabetics to wean themselves off of insulin. There are many well-documented case histories of people who have healed themselves through macrobiotic procedures.

Macrobiotics is not a religion. It is a very valuable tool that is being used to improve health, improve thinking, sharpen the senses and elevate consciousness, by thousands of individuals around the world. It utilises the same fundamentals as Feng Shui (composition in space) and 9 Ki (composition in time). But, in this case, we apply these basic principles directly to our physical bodies and our lives.

Origin

Macrobiotics has a rich and lively heritage, which originated in early Tibet and China, where three books – *The Nei Ching, The I Ching,* and *The Tao Te Ching,* largely inspired the early philosophy. The main idea propagated in these books was that humanity is part of the environment and the cosmos, and that health and judgment is a reflection of our appreciation, connection and intake from the world around us.

This diet was advocated to heal specific ailments. It also laid rule about eating. For example the food should be chewed for a longer time. Eating qualitative food to quantitative one and eating regularly in small quantities.

The Macrobiotic Diet

The word "macrobiotics" is derived from the Greek words 'Macro' and 'Bios', which mean large and life, respectively. A macrobiotic diet is one which would help a person to lead a healthy and long life. It is the science that studies the relationship between food and the environment in which we live.

This dietary pattern is also known to cure many illnesses like heart disease, cancer and diabetes.

This dietary approach of treatment can be used along with the conventional, alternative and all other forms of medicine. A macrobiotic diet should include whole grains, beans, fresh vegetables and fruits.

Food Categories and Daily Proportions under Macrobiotic Diet

Whole Cereal Grains

- 50% by weight
- Organically grown, whole grain is recommended, which can be cooked in a variety of cooking methods.
- Grains include: Brown rice, barley, millet, oats, corn, rye, wheat, and buckwheat. While whole grains are recommended, a small portion of the recommended percentage of grains may consist of noodles or pasta, un-yeasted whole grain breads, and other partially processed whole cereal grains.

Vegetables

- Approximately 20 - 30% by weight
- Local and organically grown vegetables are recommended, with the majority being cooked in various styles such as lightly steamed or boiled, sautéed with a small amount of unrefined, cold pressed oil, etc. A small portion may be used as fresh salad, and a very small volume as pickles.
- Vegetables for daily use include: green cabbage, kale, broccoli, cauliflower, collards, pumpkin, watercress, parsley, Chinese cabbage, bok choy, dandelion, mustard greens, daikon greens, scallion, onions, daikon radish, turnips, burdock, carrots, winter squash such as butternut, buttercup, and acorn squash.
- For occasional use in season (2 to 3 times a week); cucumber, celery, lettuce, herbs such as dill, chives.
- Vegetables not recommended for regular use include: eggplant, peppers, spinach, beets, and zucchini.

Beans & Sea Vegetables

- Approximately 5 - 10 % by weight
- The most suitable beans for regular use are azuki beans, chickpeas, and lentils. Other beans may be used on occasion. Bean products such as tofu, tempeh, and natto can also be used. Sea vegetables such as nori, wakame, kombu, hiziki, arame, dulse, and agar-agar form an important part of the macrobiotic diet as they provide important vitamins and minerals.

Soups

- Approximately 5 - 10 % by weight
- Soups may be made with vegetables, sea vegetables, grains, or beans. Seasonings include miso, tamari soya sauce, and sea salt.

Beverages

- Roasted bancha twig tea, stem tea, roasted brown rice tea, roasted barley tea, dandelion root tea, and cereal grain coffee.
- Any traditional tea that does not have an aromatic fragrance or a stimulating effect can also be used.

- When drinking water, spring or good quality well water is recommended, without ice.

Occasional Foods

- Fish, 1 - 3 times per week approximately 5 - 10 % by weight of that day's consumption. Recommended fish include fresh white-meat fish such as flounder, sole, cod, carp, halibut or trout.
- Fruit or fruit desserts, made from fresh or dried fruit, may be served two or three times a week. Local and organically grown fruits are preferred. If you live in a temperate climate, avoid tropical and semi-tropical fruit and instead, eat temperate climate fruits such as apples, pears, plums, peaches, apricots, berries and melons. Frequent use of fruit juice is not advisable.
- Lightly roasted nuts and seeds such as pumpkin, sesame, and sunflower seeds. Peanuts, walnuts and pecans may be enjoyed as an occasional snack.
- Rice syrup, barley malt, amasake, and mirin may be used as sweeteners.
- Brown rice vinegar or umeboshi vinegar may be used occasionally for a sour taste.

Recommended Condiments

- Gomashio, seaweed powder (kelp, kombu, wakame, and other sea vegetables), Sesame seaweed powder, umeboshi plums, tekka, pickles and sauerkraut made using sea salt, miso, or tamari.

Additional Dietary Suggestions

- Only vegetable oil should be used for cooking. To improve your health, it is preferable to use only unrefined sesame or corn oil in moderate amounts.
- Salt should be naturally processed sea salt.

Foods to Eliminate

- Meat, animal proteins, dairy products and eggs (including butter, yoghurt, ice cream, milk and cheese), refined sugars, chocolate, molasses, honey, other simple sugars and foods treated with them, and vanilla.

- Tropical or semi-tropical fruits and fruit juices, soda, artificial drinks and beverages, coffee, coloured tea, and all aromatic stimulating teas such as mint or peppermint tea.
- All artificially coloured, preserved, sprayed, or chemically treated foods. All refined and polished grains, flours, and their derivatives; mass- produced industrialized food including all canned, frozen, and irradiated foods.
- Hot spices, any aromatic stimulating food or food accessory, artificial vinegar, and strong alcoholic beverages.

(Note: Since these dietary rules are of Chinese origin, some of the elements may not be locally available. For such elements, substitutes can be used.)

Macrobiotic Lifestyle Suggestions

In order to establish a firm foundation of natural health, physiological stability and adaptability, it is vital that the following factors in our daily lives that have led to symptoms or suffering or sickness are recognised, so that we may seek or correct them. Macrobiotics is believed to be the natural cycle of life, an example of the universal rhythms of yin and yang, which occur everywhere and in everything. Macrobiotic practitioners urge you to live each day happily, without being pre-occupied with your condition, or dwelling on negative thoughts, ideas or emotions.

It is a fundamental belief that nature is essential to life, and that regular contact with nature is necessary to enjoy optimum health and well-being. There are some daily practices, which are helpful in creating a more stable and harmonious lifestyle.

- Eat only when hungry.
- Proper chewing (around 50 times or more per mouthful) is important for good digestion and assimilation of nutrients.
- Eat in an orderly and relaxed manner. When you eat, sit with a good posture and take a moment to express gratitude for the food.
- You may eat regularly two or three times per day, as much as you want, provided the proportion is generally correct and each mouthful is thoroughly chewed. It is best to leave the table satisfied but not full.

- Drink liquids moderately, only when thirsty.
- For the deepest and most restful sleep, retire before midnight and avoid eating at least 2 to 3 hours before sleeping.
- Bathe as needed but try to avoid lengthy hot baths or showers, as they can deplete the body of minerals and have a weakening effect. Preferably take brief baths or showers with a moderate temperature. If you feel fatigued after bathing you may drink a small cup of shoyubancha, or miso soup to replenish your energy.
- Use cosmetics and cleaning products that are made from natural, non-toxic ingredients. Avoid chemically perfumed products. For care of the teeth, brush with natural preparations. To maintain healthy skin function, which plays a vital part in the excretory system's regular discharging of toxins, avoid using chemically produced cosmetics and body care products. Try to use natural cosmetics from vegetable sources only.
- As much as possible, wear cotton clothing, especially for under-garments. Avoid wearing synthetic or woollen clothing directly on the skin. Avoid wearing excessive accessories on the fingers, wrists, neck, or any other part of the body.
- Spend time outdoors if strength permits. Walk on the grass, beach or soil up to one half hour every day. Spend some time in direct sunlight. Get plenty of fresh air, and when you can walk barefoot on the soil, grass or beach. Keep large green plants in your home to increase the circulation of fresh oxygen, and open windows wherever possible. It is best to use central heating and air conditioning only to the extent necessary for reasonable comfort. Allow yourself to experience the natural seasonal changes of temperature appropriate to the climate where you live.
- Exercise regularly. Activities may include walking, yoga, martial arts, dance, etc.
- Keep your home in good order, especially the areas where food is prepared and served.
- To revitalise the blood and stimulate limp circulation, scrub and massage the whole body with a hot, damp cotton towel or flannel until your skin becomes flushed, each morning or

night. At least scrub the arms, legs, hands and feet, including each finger and toe.

- Avoid using electric cooking devices such as ovens and cooking ranges or microwave oven. The use of a gas or wood stove is preferred.
- Use earthenware, cast iron, or stainless steel cookware rather than aluminium or Teflon-coated pots.
- Minimize the frequent use of television and computer display units. When using a computer, protect yourself from potentially harmful electromagnetic fields with a protective shield over the screen and other safety devices.
- Greet everyone happily and with appreciation.
- Initiate and maintain a regular correspondence with all family members, expressing thanks for their part in your life.
- Enlarge your circle of friends and acquaintances, including people from different lifestyles.
- Share your food more often by having people around; food prepared in large quantities is more satisfying and the act of sharing food is a universal gesture of human kindness and brotherhood.
- Put aside some time each day for peace and quiet, and thank your forebears and teachers for their help. Repeat your dedication to aid and support those who look to you for guidance.

The Macrobiotic Diet Pattern

Macrobiotic dietary principles are based on a simple, intuitive understanding of the body's needs and the belief that proper dietary practice is essential for the development of health, freedom and happiness.

The following principles are recommended for people who live in the world's temperate zones:

1. Each meal should be based on vegetable products with occasional supplements of animal food if necessary.
2. Whole cereal grains should constitute more than half of the meal, with occasional supplements of beans.

3. Most vegetable should be cooked rather than raw and chosen for seasonal variation. Locally grown produce is preferable to that grown at a distance and therefore out of season.
4. Sea vegetables may be used as a supplement.
5. Fruits and nuts grown in the same climate may also be used.
6. Animal food should comprise less than 15% of the meal and should always be eaten with vegetables.
7. Food should be mainly seasoned with unrefined sea salt and vegetable oil.

■■

Section Four YOUTHFUL SPIRIT

"To live is not sufficient. We need also the joy of living; and the joy of life requires health. Above all we need that health which embraces body, mind, and soul."

—Alexis Carrel

A youthful spirit has the capability of keeping the body youthful. It is the spirit and what we feel inside that is reflected on our face and body. If our spirit is pure and unadulterated, child like in purity, the body will remain free from disease and degeneration. A pure spirit is the path to happiness and true happiness keeps us young and active. A truly happy person finds joy in the very act of living; he enjoys every moment of life and is positive in outlook. Whether it is a good time or a bad time, he is able to accept both with equanimity. A happy person spreads joy all around him and dwells in a universal sense of peace and calm.

Our spirit is the most important part of the well-being. There can be no holistic health without the involvement of all factors like mind, body and spirit. To remain youthful one has to be spiritually elevated. The mind has to be cleared of all the junk that it accumulates over the years of living in a world that has many good and bad elements. Like the peeling of an onion we have to peel away the damaging thoughts and habits, layer by layer till we have reached the core which is pure and sublime. When a person is born, he is born with a clean and beautiful core; the garbage is accumulated bit by bit, over the years that are spent walking this earth. It is this garbage that we need to get rid of to achieve the clean core, in order to reach emotional well-being.

Chapter 1

CHANGING YOUR WORLD

You can change your world. I am not referring to the world that exists all around us but the one that is within each of us. If we all make an earnest effort to change that world, the external world will become a better place, eventually. The problem is that we all try to change everything around us but neglect to alter anything that is wrong with us. Ask anyone and he will tell you a hundred things that are wrong around him but ask him if everything is alright within his own self and he will not know the answer.

The solution lies in clearing up the garbage that lies within our own soul before we take a big broom and try cleaning up the society. What is the society? It is you and I; we make the society. So, how can we improve the society if we continue to be rotten inside? And believe me, we need to change not for others but for our own happiness. Cleaning up the garbage within will bring us true happiness and joy. We blame everyone and everything around us, talk of corruption and violence and of everything that is wrong with the world but we forget that it is our contribution to the world that makes all the difference.

Balancing your Needs

Maintaining psychological well-being is something of a balancing act. Firstly, you need to strike a balance between getting your own personal needs met and meeting the demands of others, both at home, at work and in the wider context of society. Secondly, you need to distribute your time and energy well, between, say, working and relaxing, or being alone and relating to others. If you devote too much time to one facet only, you not only become one-sided, but also run the risk of having no resources to fall back on in other areas when you need them. Thirdly, you have to maintain a balance between controlling and 'letting go'.

Everyone needs to be able to make and put into effect conscious choices and to have at least one area in their lives where they feel responsible and in control. But it is equally important to come to terms with the fundamental insecurity of life, its constant changeability. To be able to say goodbye, to let go, to accept chaos and 'not knowing' rather than wanting everything rigid, boxed and labelled, to be flexible and open to life and other people, these are the foundations of true peace of mind.

For many people, a belief in something larger than themselves is also an essential part of maintaining emotional balance, whether the belief is spiritual, philosophical or political. Certainly those of us whose belief structures are positive and those who find a meaning in life seem to be able to withstand its strains and stresses better.

Mind over Matter

It is now becoming more widely accepted that he mind and emotions have far greater influence on the body's state of health than was previously assumed. Most of us realise that if we feel worried or unhappy our bodies tend to feel sluggish and weary and we are more prone to aches and pains and to infections. But even those diseases that were once considered as having an exclusively 'external' origin, such as cancer, rheumatism, or heart disease, are now generally acknowledged as having a considerable psychological component. Some complementary practitioners would go even further and claim that all diseases originate in the mind, energy follows thought.

Going by the logic that there is an inter-relation between the body, mind and spirit and that they interact for the well being of the whole means that you can boost one area by positive action in another. So if you can maintain a positive, optimistic outlook, for instance, your physical health is likely to stay strong and conversely, if you improve your sense of physical well being through judicious exercise, diet and so on, your state of mind will certainly be enhanced.

A Sense of Self

Central to mental and emotional well-being is self esteem. Valuing yourself for who you are, acknowledging your own achievements, knowing your limitations, appreciating others for who they are, not for what you would like them to be, trusting your own judgement without constant reference to outside authority, these are the qualities of someone with good self-esteem. One of the foundations of self-esteem lies in having a strong sense of self, a sense of who you really are, rather than the roles you play in life. Getting in touch with this inner core enables you to see yourself as a potentially autonomous being, with the ability to shape your own life.

Changing your Beliefs

Beliefs are assumptions about reality that we hold as truths. They shape the way we act and how we feel about ourselves, but they also help to create our life experiences, since beliefs tend to be self fulfilling, if you believe you are a loser, for example, people will tend to treat you as one.

Examine your own deep beliefs about yourself and your life, and start countering some of the negative ones with creative visualisation and positive affirmations. You will find you can alter your pattern of experience and increase your sense of self.

Relating to Others

Building and nurturing good relationships with our family and friends is an essential part of emotional and physical well-being. Research studies have found that people with supportive relationships are less likely to become mentally or physically ill or suffer from accidents than those without, and that they recover more quickly from illnesses, and live longer.

We learn to relate to others from infancy onward, modelling ourselves mainly on our parents. If their relationships are fulfilling, we have a good blueprint, but relationship skills, like self-esteem, can be developed. Apart from learning to express our emotions and communicate better, we can also improve how well we relate by being more tolerant; for example, by respecting one another's privacy and difference of opinion, and by developing a sense of humour.

Positive Thinking

It is said that you can change your life through the power of positive thinking. Terminal cancer patients have sometimes recovered through this power. When the doctors give up, it is this power that takes up its place. Why else do you think that the doctors stress on the co-operation of the patient in healing. Beyond a certain point medicines have no effect·but the mind has. It transcends beyond all limits and boundaries and brings about a healing, which has not yet been explained by science.

No one really understands how or why a positive attitude helps people recover faster from surgery or cope better with serious diseases — diseases as serious as cancer, heart disease, and AIDS. But mounting evidence suggests that these effects may have something to do with the mind's power over the immune system. One recent study in the USA, for example, polled healthy first-year law students at the beginning of the school year to find out how optimistic they felt about the upcoming year. By the middle of the first semester, the students who had been confident that they would do well had more and better functioning immune cells than the worried students. Surprisingly, the students who were positive did better than the ones who didn't express optimism.

Some researchers think that pessimism may stress you out, too, boosting levels of destructive stress hormones in your bloodstream. Of course, it's also possible that having a positive attitude toward life makes you more likely to take better care of yourself. And you're more likely to attract people into your life (and keep them there) — which by itself may boost your health.

Here are some excellent tips on developing positive attitude in life.

- Find meaning in your work, daily activities, and personal relationships.
- Express anger appropriately.
- Say no to non-priorities.
- Make time for play.
- Learn from your pain and depression, and then get on with living.

- Choose healthy behaviours that meet your own needs, not someone else's ideas about what's good for you.
- Don't let outside duties keep you from meeting your basic needs. Situation Survivors remember that they are precious people first, and mothers, employees, or otherwise upstanding citizens second.

Inner Peace

Tranquillity, harmony, quietness! What does inner peace really mean? Can we buy it? Can we learn to acquire it? Does it really exist? Almost everyone muses over these questions at some time in life. Most of us consciously experience different stages in life where inner peace is more strongly experienced. People rush from one Godman to another, change from one religion to another, enlist themselves for various spiritual courses and practice all kinds of techniques to find some peace.

It seems that everyone, either consciously or sub-consciously, directly or indirectly, is seeking this elusive goal. What is it? Inner Peace is that state of being where the mind ceases to look outward, where it stops searching for things outside of itself and is content by itself. No longer does it require external factors to bring a sense of joy and happiness to it. Nothing further, especially the external, is needed.

The only way to really find inner peace is to still the outgoing mind, and to quieten the bubbling senses. Regardless of what external stimuli one can obtain, eventually one must deal with one's own restless mind. Through regular, prolonged practice of meditation and yoga *asanas* (postures), and *pranayama* (breathing exercises) one eventually gets closer to this goal. Surprisingly, it is not unlike being a better golfer, tennis player, or even a writer. One must just practice, practice, and practice. Coupled with this, one must create an atmosphere, which is conducive to more introspection and self-analysis.

Controlling Ambitions

Ambitions are a good thing. One should be ambitious because it gives a meaning and goal to life. Without ambitions, the impetus to perform better would be lost.

The question here is not whether one should be ambitious or not but how much of ambition is healthy?

There has been a sudden spurt in the ambitious nature of men and women in the last two decades. People have a constant drive to be in the fast lane, compete in the rat race and keep striving towards higher goals every moment of their life. A certain amount of stress, drive and ambition is perfectly normal; in fact it is highly desirable. But to be on a constant overdrive can be killing. This overdrive is what makes a person ruthless and uncaring. In his bid to reach the higher realm of ambitions, he stops at nothing, cares for nothing, neither about himself nor others. A highly ambitious person has no qualms about stepping on others' toes, knocking others down or neglecting his own body and soul.

We all want to do well in life, not only that we want our children to do well too. We set unrealistic targets for ourselves as well as our children leading to an unhappy family life. Unrealistic expectations mar the relationships all around us, and most of these expectations are born out of ambition.

This is dangerous. Realistic ambitions are a healthy thing but unrealistic and far-fetched ones are terribly hazardous. I have heard people say that one should aim for the sky then one can reach half way to it. But have those people ever paused to think what will occur if the person cannot even reach half way after working so hard. He will automatically suffer from frustration and anger which are a sure path to ill-health and destruction. Most of the highly ambitious persons are not healthy. They suffer from acute stress syndrome, which manifests itself in angina problems, hypertension, acidity, depression, insomnia and a host of other health problems. What is the point in being successful if you cannot enjoy the fruits of your labour because you have become so ill in the process of attaining that success? It is far better to be a little less successful and enjoy the fruits of one's labour than to strike out for more and feel the pangs of frustration.

Managing Emotions

The more we learn about the mind-body connection, the more we realise the benefits of having a control over our emotions.

Three Important Steps to Managing the Emotions

Expressing gratitude—Focusing on the positive and practicing thankfulness will crowd out those stressful negative feelings.

Have the courage to cry—Far from being a sign of weakness, shedding tears is a testimony to your inner strength.

Forgive and forget—Difficult as you may find it to seek closure; actively forgiving someone, not merely forgetting the transgression, confers countless benefits.

1. Expressing Gratitude

Seek opportunities to show appreciation for others. 'Thanks' such a simple word, and so rarely used.

- We are taught, since early childhood, to say "thank you" in response to gifts or kind gestures. Yet, in today's bustling world, we overlook the myriad opportunities to show our appreciation for others and to give back some of what we receive.
- Say "thanks" to loved ones and people you see every day. This sounds so obvious, but we tend to overlook those closest to us. It's the small things that count.

Express appreciation for people you see often and show gratitude to the community

- Clean up and weed the neighbourhood.
- Volunteer to read to children at your local library.
- Are you a computer whiz? Donate your time to a shelter and help with their computing needs.
- Donate toys, books, games and clothing to the less fortunate.
- Help an elderly lady across the street.

Show Gratitude to Yourself

- Have you ever thought of showing gratitude to yourself? After all, it is your being that is most important. Do something special for yourself, or write in your diary to reinforce your thankful attitude.
- Not only does it make others happy, but showing gratitude makes *you* feel great, too. Enjoy the benefits! Be creative!

Doing one small kindness for someone else puts a whole new perspective on your day.

2. Have the Courage to Cry

Despite society's tendency to repress emotion, expressing sadness and grief can be very therapeutic. Not only does grief take courage, but also feeling bad about any situation takes courage in our society of positive thinkers. We are bombarded by so many messages to hide our feelings, unless, of course, they are positive.

Embrace your Emotions

A phrase that people often throw around as a way of pushing their feelings aside is: "This is a learning experience." It's true that we learn from all our experiences, no matter how awful. But not everything happens to teach us a lesson. Before we can learn from sad or bad situations, we must first go through them and feel the pain. Denying our feelings only makes recovery take longer. The shame or outward denial of feeling bad begins when we are children. When youngsters are angry or depressed, we tell them to stop. Children grow through their emotions and we need to support them and allow that growth.

Tragedies and disappointments are inevitable. When we repress our feelings they come out in other self-destructive ways, including anger, rage, overeating, anorexia, drugs, alcohol, smoking or depression. It takes more courage to feel bad, and let people know how we feel, than to pretend everything is all right. If you find yourself feeling down, try a little self-talk: "A (sad, tragic, disappointing, or other appropriate word) thing happened. It is normal to feel bad, and express it. I will be more emotionally healthy and will be able to let go sooner if I feel, rather than deny."

It is also a good idea to talk to a supportive person when you have doubts about the validity of your feelings, a person who will listen and reassure you of your right to feel bad. Make sure the people you ask for support are able to give it. And finally, consider the following questions and how they relate to the experiences of your own life: How will we be able to recognise joy if we have never felt sadness? How can we know fulfilment if we have never known loss? And how can we be human if we never feel?

3. Forgive and Forget

Old resentments and failed expectations often interfere with the enjoyment of our lives — try to identify the pain and move on. Forgiveness is letting go of the need for revenge and releasing negative thoughts of bitterness and resentment. If you are a parent, you can provide a wonderful model for your children by forgiving. If they observe your reconciliation with friends or family members who have wronged you, perhaps they will learn not to harbour resentment over the ways in which you may have disappointed them. Even if you are not a parent, forgiveness is still an extremely valuable skill to have.

Forgiveness can be a gift that we give to ourselves. Here are some easy steps towards forgiveness:

- Acknowledge your own inner pain.
- Express your emotions in non-hurtful ways without yelling or attacking.
- Protect yourself from further victimisation.
- Try to understand the point of view and motivations of the person to be forgiven; replace anger with compassion.
- Forgive yourself for your role in a difficult relationship, and then decide whether or not to remain in the relationship.

Perform the overt act of forgiveness verbally or in writing. If the person you want to forgive is dead or unreachable, you can still write down your feelings in a letterform.

True Happiness

There are no simple and instant paths to happiness. It is something that needs to be worked upon. To achieve happiness, one has to work towards it. Not working as in physical labour but working as in developing a certain attitude towards life and living in general. Most of us are driven by greed and power. Power can be good and it can be bad. We generally equate power with money power, status power but never with mind power or spiritual power. The day, a person begins working towards spiritual power, he has made his way towards true happiness. Acquiring mind power and spiritual power is not as easy as acquiring money or status. It is a slow and arduous path, which demands a lot many sacrifices.

While we are working towards the greater spiritual power, we can observe some small things that will eventually add to our happiness and give us a state of contentment.

- ***Intention:*** Actively desire to be happy. Commit to happiness. Make a fully conscious decision to choose happiness over unhappiness. Once you have opted to be happy and made a commitment, it is most likely that you will try to find happiness within the same situations that existed earlier.
- ***Accountability:*** Make a choice to create the life you want to live, assume full personal responsibility for your actions, thoughts and feelings, and emphatically refuse to blame others for your own unhappiness.
- ***Identification:*** Look deeply within yourself to assess what makes you uniquely happy, apart from what others tell you about happiness. Each person has his own factors of happiness and what may make one person happy may not really make the other happy, too. You have to evaluate the elements that will constitute your happiness. Make this self-reflection a routine part of your life.
- ***Centrality:*** Insist on making what creates happiness, central in your life and make your insistence non-negotiable. When you have focussed on the central object in your life, it will be that factor that becomes prime in importance.
- ***Recasting:*** Choose to convert problems into opportunities and challenges. The ability to transform trauma into something meaningful, important and a source of emotional strength is another aspect, which will teach you to handle the adverse with equanimity.
- ***Options:*** Approach life by creating multiple scenarios. Be open to new possibilities and adopt a flexible approach to life's journey. Options give us strength and flexibility is one of the factors that go a long way towards making life far easier than an unbending attitude.
- ***Appreciation:*** Choose to deeply appreciate your life and the people in it and to stay in the present by seeing each experience as something valuable. Remember that the past never returns and you cannot undo anything, so the best thing to do is to

reflect on whatever you do. Learn to appreciate the situations that are granted to you and try to look for the positive in everything. There is always a brighter aspect to everything and detecting it can really work wonders.

- ***Giving:*** Choose to share yourself with friends and community and to give to the world at-large without the expectation of a "return." There is no greater joy than giving. When you give with an open heart, you experience contentment and happiness but when the giving is done with an expectation of a return, it loses all meaning and becomes a factor to bring discontentment and frustration because the 'return' may not materialise or suit your expectations.
- ***Truthfulness:*** Choose to be honest with yourself and to act towards others in an accountable manner by not allowing societal, corporate or family demands to violate your internal contract. It is no exaggeration that truthfulness keeps a soul clean and brings peace to the mind. A dishonest person is always insecure; he lives in fear of being discovered.
- ***Change yourself:*** Know that you can't change the world or the things around it so change your own thinking and your own self. Trying to change oneself is far better an option than trying to revolutionise and change the universe.
- ***Forgive:*** Know that to forgive you need do nothing; it is an act of the heart, not the body. Let go, give up, cease to harbour. Hoarding ill feelings and harbouring resentment causes more harm to you than to the person whom you don't want to forgive. Letting go will bring you peace and happiness.

■ ■

Chapter 2

THE PATH TO SPIRITUAL POWER

Everyone is looking for that elusive object called happiness. It is not sold in the market nor is it available in any store. It is not something that money can buy; it can be as slippery as the eel, you cannot hold on to it. There will always be the upswings and the downswings; it can't be just the ups all the time.

How many people can really claim to be happy? Most are dissatisfied and discontent with their lot, always in pursuit of something more. Happiness is not a tangible thing, it can't be seen but it has to be experienced. A pauper may be a happy soul but a prince may not be. What really is happiness? It is something people can't really explain.

A spiritual outlook could bring us closer to happiness and a feeling of joy. This joy comes from not being a rich person and having all material comforts but from the knowledge that we are closer to the almighty and are closer to self-realisation. Have you ever wondered why there is a bright radiance around the enlightened people? Why do we always paint a 'halo' around the faces of holy men and women? A halo is nothing but the radiance of pure and sublime joy around their faces.

One doesn't have to be a saint to find that joy. If we can just simplify our lives a little and improve it by a few notches, we could also find that joy. There are no prescribed paths to find the ultimate joy. One could reach there through various paths, depending on one's faith. One of the paths is that of 'meditation'. Meditation is something anyone can do. It is not difficult nor does it demand any specific conditions.

Meditation

The word 'meditation' means different things to different people. There are hundreds of different schools of mediation, many associated with some form of religious practice and many that are not. Some of these varied forms of meditation may include techniques such as complex visualisation or chanting words or sounds known as 'mantras'. Meditation is a truly holistic activity in that, ideally, the whole system of body, mind and spirit is involved and benefited.

It is the practice of concentrating on an object, word, or idea to clear the mind, relax the body, and achieve a state of heightened awareness and enlightenment. Meditation has been a feature of many religions, but it can also serve as a practical, calming therapy. It cuts off the sensory input, halts the demands of the brain, and gives the mind a chance to rest. Research projects have shown that meditation can induce relaxation, lower blood pressure, reduce the body's metabolic rate and ameliorate many stress related disorders. It is one of the greatest methods to unwind, relax the mind and trigger the body's own natural relaxation response. It is not necessary to follow the teachings of a guru or mystic to benefit from meditation.

Body

The physical benefits of mediation are easily quantifiable and plenty of research documentation exists. These include relaxation, improvement of sleeping patterns, lowering of high blood pressure, helping recovery from fatigue and general beneficial effect on most stress related disease. Posture can be helped, too, in that better posture leads to better meditation, which in turn leads to better posture. The same can be said for relaxation. The mind cannot let go until the body relaxes and vice versa.

Awareness of the body is an essential part of effective meditation. Many of the emotional stresses and upsets that people experience can be held as tensions in the body and therefore be fairly unconscious. Through the process of conscious relaxation of body and breathing that meditation entails, these stresses can be unlocked from their hiding places in the muscles and joints and simultaneously released.

Mind

Meditation teaches one to fix his mind more firmly in the present reality, to have accurate and easy recall and to make proper provisions for the future to lead a more wholesome, happy, healthy and meaningful life.

Meditation can improve the ability to concentrate, the ability to listen, both to others and yourself, and is a good way of monitoring the 'internal weather'. Although people cannot change their external conditions to any large extent, they can take the responsibility of changing their attitudes and reactions, the way the mind interacts with the world. One of the most effective and safest ways to bring about this change is to meditate. Paradoxically, meditation is not an escape from the real world; in fact, it leads to a deeper engagement with, and awareness of, one's life in order to transform it.

The forms of meditation that should be practiced, do not involve suppressing the thoughts and emotions with rigid self-control. What is required is more of a drawing together, paying ever-closer attention, becoming absorbed in your object of meditation. Meditation is not a rejection of body, neither is it a rejection of mind - specifically of thoughts. In a way, trying to stop thinking would be like trying to stop breathing. What is even more important is to change one's attitude towards these thoughts, perhaps even the nature of them, not by rigid control but by developing what might be called a feeling of inner spaciousness that can include any thought or emotion. There is then less jostling for position, less anxiety and fewer demands for attention from one's thoughts.

The path of meditation offers a way of becoming more awake and alive to every aspect, inner and outer. The mind ceases to be a burden and distraction and instead becomes a tool for paying very good attention to the present moment. The practice known as "mindfulness" is simply carrying this present – centred attention into one's daily life and activities, whether walking or running or doing household chores. In this way, meditation practice begins to become relevant to "real life" and not something separate and isolating.

Spirit

The words "spirit" and "spirituality" can be very loaded for many of us with positive and negative connotations. Those who may have suffered at the hands of dogmatic, judgemental or fundamentalist religion, may feel understandably wary of this area and reject it all together. However, spirituality may not have anything to do with any organised religion or philosophy.

Your spirituality is simply your relationship to whatever is most important or meaningful in your life – whatever nurtures you and fulfils your deepest needs. For some people this maybe money, possessions or status, but going beyond these things, ask what it is they depend on and why you need them. You may not come up with any definitive answers, but it is the asking of the questions that is important. This inquiry may lead you to discover what is truly meaningful for you; perhaps loved ones, family, home, and appreciation of beauty, honesty, a desire to discover the true meaning of life.

Proper Posture of Meditation

Generally, meditation seems to work best when the spine is straight, but relaxed and vertical. There are several reasons for this. First, sitting upright is a very good way of staying awake and alert while the eyes are closed and the attention drawn inwards. If the body is upright, the breath can begin to move in and out freely and without obstruction. Also the muscles of the torso and spine have a chance to unknot themselves of old tensions. This may not always be an entirely pain-free process. Until the body becomes used to sitting in a new more conscious way, it may fight to be allowed back to its habitual 'comfortable' state. These conflicts will pass, perhaps aided by some exercises such as yoga, tai chi or chi gung.

Eventually, proper posture will prove to be the most genuinely comfortable way of sitting still for a period of time. Sitting upright sends a message to the unconscious that although your eyes are closed; you are not going to sleep, as you would when lying down. On a more subtle level the body's Qi energy, or life force, is able to move more freely if the spine is straight. Energy cannot move through tense muscles, so a relaxed a way of sitting needs to be found.

If you find it difficult to sit on the floor, sitting in a chair is also acceptable. Given the basic requirement of an upright spine; the way of arranging the legs is a matter for personal preference and respecting the body's limits.

A major objective in the matter of posture is to ensure the free flow of breath through an open posture.

On the physical level, if the body is taking in enough breath, the brain then has sufficient oxygen to function at its peak and thus remain alert and focused. Breathing in by allowing the lower abdomen to expand enables the lungs to expand to their full extent and also relaxes the muscles of the torso and the internal organs. Many people breathe in a very shallow manner, using only their shoulders and the top part of the chest. This way of breathing can produce stress and anxiety as it provokes the 'flight-or-fight' response, meaning that rather than being alert in a relaxed and open way, they are tense and watchful. Breathing deeply, with the muscles of the abdomen relaxed, enables you to let go of deep levels of stress and tension, continuing and deepening the process of relaxation that begins with an aligned posture.

Focusing

Your breath also provides an ever present and easily accessible focus for concentration. One is always breathing! Many schools of meditation, like Vipassana, teach how to foçus on the breath in various ways.

This may involve imagining that the breath originates in one particular point of the body. The points most usually focussed on are the *hara* or *tan tien-* just below and behind the navel, or the heart, in the centre of the chest. The crown of the head, the base of the spine or the soles of the feet may all be included in the awareness. Focussing on the breath can also take the form of noticing the physical changes as the breath moves in and out, either at the nostrils or the abdomen. Meditation can be as simple as this, just breathing while sitting.

Try a simple form of meditation; find a quiet place and a comfortable sitting position that keeps your back straight. Close your eyes and concentrate on an image (a flame or flower) or on a sound or word *(mantra)* that will help clear your head of any extraneous thoughts. Breathe deeply and rhythmically, focusing attention on the chosen object or sound for 20 minutes.

There are various forms of meditation; some like Mantra meditation, Tatraka and Zazen meditation are quite popular, both in India and abroad. All methods of meditation are based on the principle of mind control, though they may use slightly different techniques. One can opt for any of the methods depending on the comfort level.

Basic Meditation

Here is another simple method to meditate. Instead of trying to memorise the method, you could make a tape for yourself and play it while meditating. This will be required only during the initial stages; once you have practised the art, it will be a very simple process.

Sitting comfortably but upright, feel your weight on the chair or cushion and relax on it. Imagine breathing in and out through your navel, taking a few deep breaths to settle in. let your attention gather at a point at the base of your spine, imagine it as a point for energy. Notice what sensations you feel there.

- Move your attention to the crown of the head, imagine a point of energy there. Notice what sensations you feel. Feel theses two points align, connected by a line of light, inside the body near though spine. Allow energy to move freely between these two points.
- Let your attention come to rest at a point of balance along this line, deep within you, at the centre of your being.
- From this centre of your being, imagine the line of light extending downward through your legs and feet, relaxing the toes and sinking into the earth. Breathing out, let all tensions and fatigue run down this line into the earth.
- Breathing in, imagine drawing up, through the soles of your feet, fresh, transformed earth energy. Allow it to fill your whole body from the feet up to the crown of your head, bringing a feeling of being supported and cradled by the solidity of the earth. Return your attention and your breathing to the centre of your being. Imagine the line of light rising to the crown of your head and above, out into the clear blue sky, to the heavens. Breathe in fresh air.

- Allow light and clearness from the heavens to radiate down the line of light to fill the whole body. Breathe into the centre of your being and feel the two energies, from the earth and the sky, mingling. From this centre let your attention be on your breath moving in and out.

■ ■

Chapter 3

CONTROLLING STRESS

Traversing through the lows and highs is a part of being. The idea is not to get defeated but to control these situations. Among the low phases of natural living, one has to deal with one more factor that has made its appearance in the last few decades. It is one of the deadliest foes that human beings have faced in the recent times and can cause enough distress to give you sleepless nights. No guesswork is required to identify that foe. It is stress I am referring to. This single word has caused enough grief to the humankind. Its stretch is wide and all encompassing, and reaches from children to elderly, making no distinction between any caste or creed. If there is any, truly, global phenomenon, it is stress. Stress is a 20th century disease but it is not likely to disappear in the next few centuries, either.

Stress

The very mention of the word 'stress' brings about anxiety and restlessness. It is something we all would like to handle better and control but most of us find it unwieldy and uncomfortable.

What is stress, and what causes it?

Stress is an inescapable part of modern life. That's the bad news. The good news is that stress isn't altogether bad news. In metered doses, it can be helpful. It can even make you better at what you do, and help give you the competitive edge. Is the major-league, non-stop, never-let-up stress you have to watch out for. Because, it can kill you.

Stress is an adaptive response. It's the body's reaction to an event that is seen as emotionally disturbing, disquieting, or threatening. When we perceive such an event, we experience what one stress researcher called the "fight or flight" response. To prepare for fighting or fleeing, the body increases its heart rate and blood pressure; more blood is then sent to your heart and muscles, and your respiration rate increases. This response was probably beneficial to our cavemen ancestors who had to fight off wild animals. But today, stress itself has become the "wild animal." Untamed and allowed to run rampant in our lives, it can destroy our health. Not only is uncontrolled stress harmful to our bodies but it can also lead to unwise behaviours such as alcohol and drug abuse, which place us at even greater risk, health wise. It can also jeopardise our relationships, by leading to emotional outbursts and, in some cases, physical violence.

Life without stimulus would be incredibly dull and boring. Life with too much stimulus becomes unpleasant and tiring, and may ultimately damage your health or well-being. Too much stress can seriously interfere with your ability to perform effectively and a consistently high level of stress over a sustained period can damage your health.

The art of stress management is to keep yourself at a level of stimulation that is healthy and enjoyable. Most people realise that aspects of their work and lifestyle can cause stress. While this is true, it is also important to note that it can be caused by your environment and by the food and drink you consume. There are several major sources of stress:

- ***Survival Stress:*** this may occur in cases where your survival or health is threatened, where you are put under pressure, or where you experience some unpleasant or challenging event. Here adrenaline is released in your body and you experience all the symptoms of your body preparing for 'fight or flight'.
- ***Internally generated stress:*** this can come from anxious worrying about events beyond your control, from a tense, hurried approach to life, or from relationship problems caused by your own behaviour. It can also come from an 'addiction' to and enjoyment of stress.

- ***Environmental and Job stress:*** here your living or working environment causes the stress. It may come from noise, crowding, pollution, untidiness, dirt or other distractions. Alternatively stress can come from events at work.
- ***Fatigue and overwork:*** here stress builds up over a long period. This can occur where you try to achieve too much in too little time, or where you are not using effective time management strategies.

Of all the stressors, the ones related to lifestyle and jobs are the most common. In fact, they form the bulk of stressors. Let us have a look at some of them; it will help you to identify these stressors and learn to deal with them.

Lifestyle and Job Stress

Many of the stresses you experience may come from your job or from your lifestyle. These may include:

Job Related Stress

- Too much or too little work
- Having to perform beyond your experience or perceived abilities
- Having to overcome unnecessary obstacles
- Time pressures and deadlines
- Keeping up with new developments
- Changes in procedures and policies
- Lack of relevant information, support and advice lack of clear objectives unclear expectations of your role from your boss or colleagues responsibility for people, budgets or equipment.

Career Development Stress

- Under-promotion, frustration and boredom with current role
- Over-promotion beyond abilities
- Lack of a clear plan for career development
- Lack of opportunity
- Lack of job security

Personal and Family Stresses

- Financial problems

- Relationship problems
- Ill-health
- Family changes such as birth, death, marriage or divorce.

Stress Symptoms

Stress may manifest itself through various symptoms, which can be divided into three categories –

1. Emotional Symptoms
2. Behavioural Symptoms
3. Physical Symptoms

1. Emotional Symptoms of Stress

Stress causes many complaints and conditions. When one or more of these signs or symptoms occur more frequently than normal, or are more difficult to shrug off, it indicates that your stress level is becoming unacceptably high. And it is time to review your lifestyle and take steps to reduce stress.

- Worry or anxiety
- Confusion and inability to concentrate or make decisions
- Feeling ill
- Feeling out of control or overwhelmed by events
- Frequent mood changes:
- Depression
- Frustration
- Hostility
- Helplessness
- Impatience and irritability
- Restlessness
- Being more lethargic
- Difficulty in sleeping
- Drinking more alcohol and smoking
- Changing eating habits
- Reduced sex drive
- Relying more on medication

2. Behavioural Symptoms of Stress

Stress influences behaviour. When you or other people are under pressure, this can show as:

- Talking too fast or too loud
- Yawning
- Fiddling and twitching, nail biting, grinding teeth, drumming fingers, pacing, etc.
- Being irritable
- Defensiveness
- Being critical
- Aggression
- Irrationality
- Overreaction and reacting emotionally

Reduced Personal Efficiency

- Being unreasonably negative
- Making less realistic judgements
- Being unable to concentrate and having difficulty making decisions
- Being more forgetful
- Making more mistakes
- Being more accident prone
- Changing work habits
- Increased absenteeism
- Neglect of personal appearance

These symptoms of stress should not be taken in isolation - other factors could cause them. However if you find yourself exhibiting or recognising a number of them, then it would be worth investigating your levels of stress.

3. Physical Symptoms of Stress

The physical symptoms can be of two kinds – the short-term symptoms and the long-term symptoms.

Short Term Physical Symptoms

These mainly occur as your body adapts to perceived physical threat, and are caused by release of adrenaline. Although you may perceive these as unpleasant and negative, they are signs that your body is ready for the explosive action that assists survival or high performance:

- Faster heart beat
- Increased sweating
- Cool skin
- Cold hands and feet
- Feelings of nausea, or 'Butterflies in stomach'
- Rapid Breathing
- Tense Muscles
- Dry Mouth
- A desire to urinate
- Diarrhoea

While adrenaline helps you survive in a 'fight-or-flight' situation, it does have negative effects in situations where this is not the case because it interferes with clear judgement and makes it difficult to take the time to make good decisions.

Effects of Short term physical stress

- Where you need good physical skills it gets in the way of fine motor control.
- It causes difficult situations to be seen as a threat, not a challenge.
- It damages the positive frame of mind you need for high quality work by:
    - Promoting negative thinking,
    - Damaging self-confidence,
    - Narrowing attention,
    - Disrupting focus and concentration and
    - Making it difficult to cope with distractions
- It consumes mental energy in distraction, anxiety, frustration and temper. This is energy that should be devoted to the work in hand.

Long Term Physical Symptoms

These occur where your body has been exposed to adrenaline over a long period. One of the ways adrenaline prepares you for action is by diverting resources to the muscles from the areas of the body, which carry out body maintenance. This means that if you are exposed to adrenaline a sustained period, then your health may start to deteriorate. This may show up in several ways like:

- Change in appetite
- Frequent colds
- Asthma
- Back pain
- Digestive problems
- Headaches
- Skin eruptions
- Sexual disorders
- Aches and pains
- Feelings of intense and long-term tiredness

Assessing your Stress Level

At some time in your life there will be some incident or event that causes major stress and may alter your lifestyle. Such crises are often known as life events. Emotional trauma caused by divorce, bereavement and moving house are stressful life events. Researchers discovered that our adaptability and ability to relax and cope with stress was damaged when we go through prolonged period of stressful life events in a single year. Some people find one particular life event more damaging than another; heredity, lifestyle and diet all affect and individual's response to stress.

Optimal Stress

There is no single level of stress that is optimal for all people. We are all individual creatures with unique requirements. As such, what is distressing to one may be a joy to another. And even when we agree that a particular event is distressing, we are likely to differ in our physiological and psychological responses to it. The person who loves to arbitrate disputes and moves from job site to job site would be stressed in a job, which was stable, and routine, whereas the person who thrives under stable conditions would very likely be stressed on a job when duties were highly varied. Also, our personal stress requirements and the amount which we can tolerate before we become distressed, changes with our age.

It has been found that most illness is related to unrelieved stress. If you are experiencing stress symptoms, you have gone beyond your optimal stress level; you need to reduce the stress in your life and/or improve your ability to manage it.

Elimination of Stress

A stress free existence is, perhaps, a mirage. The pressures of modern living ensure that stress is always lurking in the background. It can not be eliminated but one could try to control it.

Stress can be good and bad, depending on the type. Positive stress adds anticipation and excitement to life, and we all thrive under a certain amount of stress. Deadlines, competitions, confrontations, and even our frustrations and sorrows add depth and enrichment to our lives. Our goal is not to eliminate stress but to learn how to manage it and how to use it to help us. Insufficient stress acts as a depressant and may leave us feeling bored or dejected; on the other hand, excessive stress may leave us feeling "tied up in knots." What we need to do is find the optimal level of stress, which will individually motivate but not overwhelm each of us.

Managing Stress

Identifying unrelieved stress and being aware of its effect on our lives is not sufficient for reducing its harmful effects. Just as there are many sources of stress, there are many possibilities for its management. However, the best among them is changing the source of stress and changing your reaction to it.

Be aware of your stressors and your reactions.

Notice your distress. Don't ignore it. Don't gloss over your problems. Determine what events distress you. What are you telling yourself about meaning of these events? Determine how your body responds to the stress. Do you become nervous or physically upset? If so, in what specific ways?

Ask Yourself -

- Are you a perfectionist?
- Do you feel a constant pressure to achieve?
- Do you criticise yourself when you are not perfect?
- Do you feel you haven't done enough no matter how hard you try?
- Do you give up pleasure in order to be the best in everything you do?
- Does your self-esteem depend on everyone else's opinion of you?
- Do you sometimes avoid assignments because you're afraid of disappointing your boss?
- Are you better at caring for others than caring for yourself?
- Do you keep most negative feelings inside to avoid displeasing others?

If the answer to all these questions is a 'yes', then you are a victim of stress.

Recognise what you can change

Can you change your stressors by avoiding or eliminating them completely? Can you reduce their intensity and manage them over a period of time instead of on a daily or weekly basis? Shorten your exposure to stress, take a break, and relax.

Can you devote the time and energy necessary to making a change? goal setting, time management techniques, and delayed gratification strategies may be helpful here.

You cannot change everything but there are three things you can change– your thinking, your behaviour and your lifestyle.

Change Your Thinking

- Practice reframing of thoughts
- Use the power of Positive thinking

Change Your Behaviour

- Be Assertive
- Get Organized/ learn the technique of Time Management
- Express your feelings (ventilate)

- Develop a strong sense of humour
- Pick up some hobby

Change Your Lifestyle

- Take healthy diet
- Exercise regularly
- Drink gallons of water
- Keeping a pet can be therapeutic
- Try Meditation
- Deep Breathing relieves stress
- Nature Walks and Imagery are extremely useful
- Practice the magic of Hydrotherapy: A Warm, Hot Bath
- Indulge in soulful Music Therapy
- Grab enough sleep
- Make time for leisure

Reduce the intensity of your emotional reactions to stress

The stress reaction is triggered by your perception of danger. Are you viewing your stressors in exaggerated terms and/or taking a difficult situation and making it a disaster? Are you expecting to please everyone?

Are you overreacting and viewing things as absolutely critical and urgent? Do you feel you must always prevail in every situation? Work at adopting more moderate views; try to see the stress as something you can cope with rather than something that overpowers you. Try to temper your excess emotions. Put the situation in perspective. Do not labour on the negative aspects and the "what if..." imagination.

Learn to moderate your physical reactions to stress

Slow, deep breathing will bring your heart rate and respiration back to normal.

Relaxation techniques can reduce muscle tension. Electronic biofeedback can help you gain voluntary control over such things as muscle tension, heart rate, and blood pressure.

Medications, when prescribed by a physician, can help in the short term in moderating your physical reactions. However, they alone are not the answer. Learning to moderate these reactions on your own is a preferable long-term solution.

Build your physical reserves

Exercise for cardiovascular fitness three to four times a week (moderate, prolonged rhythmic exercise is best, such as walking, swimming, cycling, or jogging). Eat well-balanced, nutritious meals. Maintain your ideal weight. Avoid nicotine, excessive caffeine, and other stimulants. Mix leisure with work. Take breaks and get away when you can. Get enough sleep. Be as consistent with your sleep schedule as possible.

Maintain your emotional reserves

Develop some mutually supportive friendships/relationships. Pursue realistic goals, which are meaningful to you, rather than goals others have for you that you do not share. Expect some frustrations, failures, and sorrows. Always be kind and gentle with yourself—be a friend to yourself.

Get organised

Although it is a waste of energy to worry about future events over which we have no control, it is human nature to do so. Plan and prioritise as best you can, and then be easy on yourself. The future has not happened, and the past is not going to happen again.

Time Management

One of the most common causes of stress is being disorganized at work or at home. Here are some tips to get organized. Keep a diary. Write lists of tasks to accomplish prioritise them and schedule when you will complete them.

Writing down objectives, duties and activities helps to make them more tangible and workable. Having a schedule also helps you provide the facts when your boss asks you to perform unreasonable tasks. They may have no idea that you are overwhelmed with work and the additional responsibilities cannot be accomplished unless something else goes. Again, prioritising tasks helps you to minimize the stressful situations.

Make a List and Prioritise

So many projects, so little time. To beat stress, you have to learn to prioritise. At the start of each day, pick the single most important task to complete, and then finish it. If you're a person who makes to-do lists, never write one with more than five items. That way, you're more likely to get all the things done, and you'll feel a greater sense of accomplishment and control. Then you can go ahead and make a second five-item list. While you're at it, make a list of things that you can delegate to co-workers and family members.

Learn To Say 'No' When Appropriate

Sometimes you have to learn to draw the line. Stressed-out people often can't assert themselves. Instead of saying 'I don't want to do this' or 'I need some help,' they do it all themselves. Then they have even more to do."

Give your boss a choice. Say 'I'd really like to take this on, but I can't do that without giving up something else. Which of these things would you like me to do?' Most bosses can take the hint. The same strategy works at home, with your spouse, children, relatives and friends.

If you have trouble-saying 'no', start small. Tell your hubby to make his own sandwich. Or tell your daughter to reach home on her own, after her music class. Pad your schedule. Realise that nearly everything will take longer than you anticipate. By allotting yourself enough time to accomplish a task, you cut back on anxiety. In general, if meeting deadlines is a problem, always give yourself 20 percent more time than you think you need to do the task.

Ventilation

People who keep things for themselves without sharing with their friends or loved ones carry a considerable and unnecessary burden. Share your problems and concern with others. Develop a support system of relatives, colleagues or friends to talk to when you are upset or worried. When you are frustrated write it down. After you have vent the frustration, destroy the writing so that it is forgotten. Re-reading the journal will reawaken the frustration and anger. So, do not keep it.

Seek social support. Studies have shown that close, positive relationships with others facilitate good health and morale. One reason for this is that support from family and friends serves as a buffer to cushion the impact of stressful events. Talking out problems and expressing tensions can be incredibly helpful.

Relaxation

Stress and relaxation are two sides of the same coin and both are necessary for a healthy life. When they are in balance all is well, but if stress predominates, illness often develops – the possible consequences can range from headaches, anxiety and lethargy to heart attacks, ulcers or cancer. While experts agree that stress plays a part in the onset of many disorders, it is also an accepted truth that not all stress is bad. Even events like getting married, receiving a promotion, having a baby are stressful, but good for you. All stress comes from two basic sources: physical activity and mental or emotional activity.

Emotional frustration is more likely to cause stress-related disease, such as ulcers, than any type of physical work, though overwork accompanied by failure or lack of purpose can lead to exhaustion and even breakdown. However, the absence of work is no cure, and being excessively relaxed and indifferent to stress would mean missing out on all the wonderful feelings that add spice to life: euphoria, for example; excitement; heightened awareness of sounds, colour and smells; exhilaration; a sense of triumphing over the odds; and the heady scent of success. A well-adjusted approach to life's inherent pressures implies the juggling of all kinds of stress-both positive and negative – in order to achieve the balance we strive for.

Stress Management Techniques

Almost every day, a new method is being invented or re-discovered. Almost any method that can lighten your mind is effective, if practiced regularly.

Stress management can be done through **mental** and **physical** techniques. Mental techniques includes various methods like meditation, Pranayam, imagery, self hypnosis, Reiki, Vipassana etc. while physical methods are mainly to do with physical exercises of various kinds e.g. aerobics, Tai chi etc.

Choosing a Technique

To many people, relaxation does not come naturally, though stress does. Because of this, most people have to make a special effort to learn how to relax. Each individual must choose from the combination of the techniques that are available, until you find those that suit you and your lifestyle; when you try any particular one, concentrate on what you personally want out of it, and remember that you are more likely to succeed if you choose a method and stick to it.

Some of the techniques described have primarily a mental effect; others mainly affect the body. Many of the mental techniques originate in the East, where they have been used for centuries to achieve deep relaxation, inner peace and tranquillity. If you feel that such qualities are missing in your life try one of these techniques – meditation, for example.

Other techniques are based on achieving a physical harmony and balance that will, in turn, affect mental well-being. If you find it easier to achieve physical and mental relaxation through movement or 'doing something', these are the techniques for you.

Whichever techniques you choose, persevere with them for a while before trying another one, quick changes are in themselves a sign of stress.

1. Basic Relaxation Technique

A self-help technique to reduce accumulated stress in the body, by progressively contracting and relaxing the muscle groups that store tension. While it is essential that our muscles maintain a certain amount of tension to support posture and movement, it is when our bodies have to move unnaturally or under stress that the result can be extra, unnecessary tension in certain muscles – for example, in neck and shoulders. This itself causes symptoms of stress- headaches, aches and pains and general tiredness, for example- and so the vicious circle is established.

To break out of this circle we need to know how to release excess tension from the muscles – this is the first step in relaxation, and is used in all the various techniques. To succeed, however, one important lesson should be borne in mind; that is, a recognition that most of the time we tend to concentrate on what is happening in the outside world around us, whereas the essence of relaxation is to bring that focus back inside ourselves, so that we may become sensitive to the tensions within and begin to relieve them.

Put on loose, comfortable clothes, making sure that your feet are warm.

- Lie down in a quiet, warm, dark room, using the floor, a mat or a firm bed – this is perhaps the best position for a beginner, though alternative positions are given below. Place a pillow or cushion under your head and knees. Either let your hands and arms rest by your side or gently upon your stomach, whichever feels the most comfortable.
- Check that you feel really comfortable. If necessary, use more pillows – perhaps under your feet and forearms. Only start the technique once you are certain of your comfort.
- Relax and let your mind go blank. Take a couple of deep breaths and sigh the air away.
- Now you are ready to start reducing tension in your muscles. The technique involves letting go of all the muscles in the body, starting at the toes, working gradually up the body and ending with the face. To begin, concentrate on your left foot. Tense all the muscles – curling the toes and scrunching the foot. Hold for a few seconds. Let go, and make them feel floppy, heavy and warm, as if they are sinking in to the pillow. It may take a little practice to perfect this technique, but it will come if you persevere.
- Move onto the calf muscles on the left leg. Tense the muscles, hold and let go. Feel the heaviness and warmth of the leg and foot.
- Apply the same technique on the left thigh. Concentrate on the left leg – does it feel heavy, warm, and relaxed. Is it sinking into the floor or bed? If the answers are 'no', tense the whole leg, hold it in tension until it feels difficult to hold the position any longer, then let go completely.
- Repeat the same process with the right leg.
- When both legs feel heavy and numb, continue moving up the body. Clench your buttocks tightly and let go; pull in your stomach muscles, hold tight, relax; let them fallback towards the spine into the floor or bed. Feel the warmth spreading up your body.

- Breathe deeply and evenly a few times, then sigh the breath away; imagine you are sighing all the tension out of your body.
- Move on to your left hand, squeeze your hand into a fist, hold tight and let go. Tighten the muscles in the arm, let them flop. Continue with your right arm. Repeat if the arms are not relaxed and heavy. They should feel numb and impossible to move.
- Hunch your shoulders up towards your ears, hold, let go; let them sink into the floor. It may be necessary to repeat this movement a few times as we hold a lot of tension in our shoulders. Pull the shoulders up towards the ceiling and let them flop back into the ground. Repeat a couple of times.
- Rock your head gently from side to side in order to loosen the neck. Feel the total relaxation of the body and breathe deeply a few times. Relax, feel the warmth and quiet,
- The face is the most difficult part of the body to relax; yawn widely with an open mouth, let go; purse the lips out in a pout, then relax; frown fiercely, let go; move the scalp by raising the eyebrows, then relax.
- The whole body should now be relaxed. Breathe evenly in and out, saying to yourself with each breath that you feel more and more relaxed, peaceful and warm.
- Rest, relaxed and warm for around 15 minutes. Do not jump up and start racing around. Let yourself come to slowly and gently; stretch and give yourself a shake before allowing the outside world to impinge on your mind.

2. Shavasana – The Ultimate Relaxation Technique

There is no doubt that there are many techniques of stress control that are being practised by people in the present times. But one technique that remains unbeatable is the yogic shavasana.

Complete relaxation is a combination of physical state and the mental state. It is the physical state when the muscles are soft and without tension and the brain waves slow down to a serene state of emotional and mental calm. This is the Alpha state in which the brain's rhythm slows down to 8-14 cycles per second and the two halves of the brain are in balance. In this state the immune system is working at its optimum level and the body is able to heal itself easily. The mind is at its peak, both creatively and intuitively. This is the state of ultimate relaxation or deep relaxation, as it is called.

Shavasana is the prelude to reaching the Alpha state, which is the key to good health, creative thinking and intuition. It is equivalent to the Zen 'No Mind' state, a state where you are in touch with the deeper levels of the mind. Anyone can reach that state through the practice of shavasana. All one requires is a peaceful place and an ability to loosen the mind. Shavasana, which literally means 'Dead Man's Pose', is an effective way to let go of the physical and mental tensions.

- Lie flat on your back with the hands resting alongside. Keep the legs straight and together with the heels touching each other.
- Relax all the muscles in the body. Begin with the toes and loosen up the muscles till they become limp. Next, release the muscles of the ankles progressing upwards slowly to the calves and then the thighs. As you traverse through each part of the body keep relaxing the muscles groups in that area. Loosen up the muscles in the hips, abdomen, heart, the shoulders, neck, arms, elbows and the palm till you reach the fingers. Finally, let the muscles of the head, eyes, lips and ears be relaxed.
- By the time you have finished with all the muscles in the body, you will begin to experience a feeling of total relaxation and your breathing will have slowed down to become more regular.
- Lie in this pose for about five minutes, turn to the left and count 12, next turn to the right and count 12. Now get up slowly from your right side.

Initially, you could begin with holding the position for about 5 minutes and then increase the duration to 15 minutes, gradually.

This asana is excellent for hypertension and blood pressure relief.

Relaxation Checklist

Once you have mastered the relaxation techniques, you can apply them almost anywhere. It is important, though, to cultivate an awareness of how your body feels throughout the day, so that you can learn to recognise the difference between normal and unnatural amounts of tension. Once you begin to notice when and where you tense up, you can pinpoint your exercises to relax those muscle groups that are affected.

- Don't leap out of bed in the morning late, with too much to do before you start the day. Set the alarm just 5 minute earlier to give yourself time to relax.
- Plan to have time to yourself at home – when the children are at school, for example, or playing peacefully. Let the family know that certain times of the day are 'your time' – then lie down or sink into a chair and empty your mind of all household and work problems. Concentrate on how your body feels and note areas of tension; then use the relaxation technique.
- Watch out for tension in your shoulders and arms when driving a car. Are you gripping the steering wheel, sitting bolt upright and frowning? At traffic lights or in a traffic jam, take a few seconds to concentrate on yourself; hunch the shoulders up, then let them flop down; slacken your grip on the steering wheel; relax back into your seat and feel the tension leave your body. Breathe slowly and deeply – it is difficult to become angry and frustrated while you are doing this.

■ ■

Chapter 4

BREATHING HEALTHY

The importance of correct breathing has been recognised since beginning of history. The Shaman, the wise men and witch doctors of ancient times, used breathing techniques to induce trances or to improve performance. Correct breathing was and still is considered to be vital for good health, in eastern medicine. It is also thought to be essential if one is to progress to the higher levels of skills in meditational and martial arts and in the achievement of the 'asanas' or postures taken up during T'ai Chi and yoga exercise, for example. Today, it is generally recognised that correct breathing has an important role to play, in particular, in helping to reduce levels of stress as well as its signs and symptoms.

The environmental strains of modern urban life have made breathing techniques even more important than they have been in the past since the air that we take in to our bodies is polluted with smoke and chemicals that can damage lung tissues. Polluted air is dangerously low in oxygen – vital for the physical and the mental health of the body – and low in the atmospheric ions that are linked with positive health.

Since it is impractical for the majority of us to start a new life in the less polluted countryside, it is vitally important that we breathe as efficiently as possible.

Importance of Breathing

Breathing is important for two reasons. It is the only means to supply our bodies and its various organs with the supply of oxygen, which is vital for our survival. The second function of breathing is that it is one means to get rid of waste products and toxins from the body.

During inspiration (breathing in), air is drawn into the lungs, where it fills tiny air sacs that are surrounded by a network of miniscule blood vessels. The blood then absorbs the oxygen and transports it around the body to supply every cell. As the oxygen is absorbed, the blood passes carbon di-oxide- the waste product of energy released from the cells-back into the air, to be removed from the body during expiration (breathing out).

Though we all breathe by instinct, most people only use only about half their lung capacity, the result being that the air sacs (alveoli) absorb too little oxygen, leaving an excess of carbon di oxide in the tissues which is reabsorbed by the blood. Conversely, panic or anxiety attacks, when breathing can become so shallow and rapid; a condition known as hyperventilation – that the body expels too much carbon di oxide, are a problem for some people. With practice, though, breathing can be made more efficient, so that hyperventilation during anxiety can be avoided by controlled breathing, thereby reducing stress and leading to general well being.

Vital Oxygen

Oxygen is the most vital nutrient for our bodies. It is essential for the integrity of the brain, nerves, glands and internal organs. We can do without food for weeks and without water for days, but without oxygen, we will die within a few minutes. If the brain does not get proper supply of this essential nutrient, it will result in the degradation of all vital organs in the body.

The brain requires more oxygen than any other organ. If it doesn't get enough, the result is mental sluggishness, negative thoughts and depression and, eventually, vision and hearing decline.

Yogis realised the vital importance of an adequate oxygen supply thousands of years ago. They developed and perfected various breathing techniques. These breathing exercises are particularly important for people who have sedentary jobs and spend most of the day in offices. Their brains are oxygen starved and their bodies are just 'getting by'. They feel tired, nervous and irritable and are not very productive. On top of that, they sleep badly at night, so they get a bad start to the next day, continuing the cycle. This situation also lowers their immune system, making them susceptible to catching colds, flu and other infections.

Secret of Vitality

One of the major secrets of vitality and rejuvenation is a purified blood stream. The quickest and most effective way to purify the blood stream is by taking in extra supplies of oxygen from the air we breathe. The breathing exercises described in here are the most effective methods ever devised for saturating the blood with extra oxygen. By purifying the blood stream, every part of the body as well as the mind benefits. Your complexion will become clearer and brighter and wrinkles will begin to fade away. In short, rejuvenation will begin to occur.

Scientists have known for a long time that there exists a strong connection between respiration and mental states. Improper breathing produces diminished mental ability. It is known that mental tensions produce restricted breathing. A normally sedentary person, when confronted with a perplexing problem, tends to lean forward, draw his arms together, and bend his head down. All these body postures result in reduced lung capacity.

We become fatigued from the decreased circulation of the blood and from the decreased availability of oxygen for the blood because we have almost stopped breathing. As our duties and responsibilities become more demanding, we develop habit of forgetting to breathe.

Incorrect Breathing

Our breathing is too shallow and too quick. We are not taking in sufficient oxygen and we are not eliminating sufficient carbon dioxide. As a result, our bodies are oxygen starved, and a toxic build-up occurs.

Shallow breathing does not exercise the lungs enough, so they lose some of their function, causing a further reduction in vitality. Animals, which breathe slowly, live the longest; the elephant is a good example.

We need to breathe more slowly and deeply. Quick shallow breathing results in oxygen starvation which leads to reduced vitality, premature ageing, poor immune system and a myriad of other factors. Shallow breathing also results in reduced vitality, since oxygen is essential for the production of energy in the body, and increased disease. Our resistance to disease is reduced, since oxygen is essential for healthy cells. This means we catch more colds and develop other ailments more easily.

Correct Breathing

Start by learning correct breathing techniques when lying down, alone and without distractions. Once you have mastered the technique, it can be practiced in any position, anywhere – eventually it will become a habit.

1. Wear loose, comfortable clothes and lie on your back on the floor using a mat, or on your bed.
2. Place both your hands on the lower edges of your ribs, with fingers nearly touching.
3. Relax your body.
4. Breathe in deeply and smoothly through your nostrils. Feel your diaphragm pulling out and down, your stomach rising and your ribs expanding upwards and outwards. Hold the breath for a few seconds.
5. Breathe out smoothly. This requires no muscular activity, since all that happens is that the diaphragm and the muscles of the chest let go, but try to ensure that all the air that you inhaled is expelled. The ribs collapse down and in; the stomach lowers.
6. Repeat three or four times, then relax and breathe naturally for a few minutes, before starting the sequence once again.

Note:

- Your shoulders should remain stationary during breathing. Many people, especially women breathe solely into their upper lobes by raising and lowering their shoulders. This does not give the body an adequate supply of oxygen and is a common symptom of stress.
- If you feel heady and faint during the breathing exercises, relax and breathe naturally for a few minutes – the sensation passes quickly and is the result of the brain receiving an unusually large amount of oxygen.

Breathing While Sitting

1. Make sure you are sitting comfortable with your spine straight.
2. Relax your shoulders and place your hands loosely on your lap.
3. Breathe using the same basic method as for lying down.
4. Feel the air filling your lungs, right down to the bottom lobes.
5. Check your shoulders – they should not be moving up and down.
6. If you feel that you are not filling your lungs fully, place your hands on the bottom edge of the ribs, and over the stomach and check that your ribs and stomach are expanding fully under your fingers as you breathe in. Breathe in this manner a few times until you sense the movement and then return your hands to your lap.

Breathing While Walking

1. Walk at a steady pace, letting your hands swing loosely by your side.
2. Breathe in deeply – as in the basic method- for a certain number of paces, hold the breath for half that number and breathe out gradually for the same number. Find which number of paces feels right for you.
3. Maintain the rhythm and repeat the exercise five times. Then relax and breathe naturally.
4. Repeat the whole exercise a few times during each walk.

The Healing Breath

This method of healing in used in all branches of eastern medicine, though not in orthodox western medicine. It involves breathing in the *chi*, as Chinese and Japanese medicine calls the 'life force', or the *prana*, as Indian medicine names it, into the lungs and visualising it flowing from them first into the solar plexus and then to the area to be healed. During exhalation the disease is visualised flowing out of the body.

The Re-energising Breath

These two exercises in breathing will first perform a releasing function on your body and mind and then re-charge them. The second exercise is especially structured to boost your vitality but it should be used sparingly to prevent hyperventilation.

- Breathe in deeply through an open mouth and sigh out with a relaxed throat. Your upper back widens on inhale, and releases on exhale. Don't worry if you yawn; it's your body's homeostatic mechanism correcting your oxygen and carbon dioxide balance.
- Open your mouth wide, inhale deeply and let the air out in a big 'hah'. Repeat a few times quickly. If you feel light-headed, breathe normally through your nose. Tingling in your mouth or fingers is a normal reaction to shifting levels of oxygen and carbon dioxide.

Tension Reliever

This exercise is particularly useful, since it only takes a few minutes and can be performed anywhere, at any time.

1. Stand up with your hands hanging loosely by your side.
2. Breathe in slowly through your nostrils, tensing all your muscles at the same time.
3. Hunch your shoulders up to your ears, clench your hands as hard as possible, tighten your stomach muscles, clench your buttocks and raise yourself up on to tiptoe.
4. Hold this position to the count of five. Fix your eye on something straight ahead to help you balance.
5. Slowly breathe out through your nostrils and at the same time relax all your muscles, so that by the time you have fully exhaled your shoulders are down, your hands are floppy, your stomach is relaxed and your knees are slightly bent.
6. Repeat five times.

Alternate Nose Breathing

This breathing technique is recommended for calming the spirit and the mind. The sun and moon are seen here as symbols of the positive and negative, and this technique shows you how to inhale the positive energy of the sun and exhale the negative waste products of the body.

1. Sit in an upright position – cross-legged if you can manage it, otherwise sit on a firm backed chair.

2. Pinch your nostrils shut with your right hand, the thumb closing the right nostril and the index and middle finger closing the left nostril. Only gentle pressure is needed, so do not pinch too hard.
3. Breathe through your mouth as you practise opening and closing the nostrils alternately.
4. When you have learnt how to do this, inhale deeply and slowly as for the basic method through your right nostril – keep the left nostril firmly closed.
5. Hold for the amount of time it took you to inhale – tough not if it feels uncomfortable.
6. Exhale gradually through your left nostril again for the same length of time it took to inhale. The comparative ratio for these three motions – breathing in, holding, then breathing out – is therefore 1:1:1. This rhythm can take a while to master, but the control it engenders and the results are worthwhile. Traditionally, those advanced in yoga use a ratio of 1:4:2, but without specialised training you should not try to go beyond 1:2:2.
7. Breathe in this way five times and then use the left nostril to inhale and the right nostril to exhale and repeat.
8. Breathe twice through both nostrils deeply and fully.
9. Relax totally in the same position and feel the tension disappearing.

The De-stressing Breath

The more stressed out we are, the tighter we hold ourselves, especially in the jaw, chest and diaphragm. If we breathe deeply, the oxygen flows, and we can think and feel more clearly.

This exercise will help you de-stress and unwind.

- Sit cross-legged on the floor, or in a chair with your feet flat on the ground, head straight and chin parallel to the floor.
- Inhale slowly through your nose, filling your abdomen, ribs and chest. Then blow out steadily though puckered lips until your lungs are empty.
- Breathe in again, feeling your torso muscles move like a bellows. Imagine expelling tension from your body.

Pranayama: The Breathing Exercises of Yoga

Pranayama, as traditionally conceived, involves much more than merely breathing for relaxation. Pranayama is a term with a wide range of meanings. Patanjali defines pranayama as "the regulation of the incoming and outgoing flow of breath with retention." It is to be practiced only after perfection in asana is attained. Pranayama also denotes cosmic power, or the power of the entire universe, which manifests itself as conscious living being in us through the phenomenon of breathing.

The word pranayama consists of two parts: prana and ayama.

Prana is energy, when the self-energising force embraces the body. When this self-energising force embraces the body with extension, expansion and control, it is pranayama.

Prana is an auto-energising force which creates a magnetic field in the form of the Universe and plays with it, both to maintain and to destroy for further creation. It acts as physical energy, mental energy, where the mind gathers information; and as intellectual energy, where information is examined and filtered. Prana also acts as sexual energy, spiritual energy and cosmic energy. All that vibrates in this Universe is prana: heat, light, gravity, magnetism, vigour, power, vitality, electricity, life and spirit are all forms of prana. It is the cosmic personality, potent in all beings and non-beings. It is the prime mover of all activity. It is the wealth of life.

Ayama means stretch, extension, expansion, length, breadth, regulation, prolongation, restraint and control and describes the action of pranayama.

Importance of Healthy Breathing

We know how to breathe. It is something that occurs to us automatically, spontaneously, naturally. We are breathing even when we are not aware of it. So it seems foolish to think that one can be told how to breathe. Yet, one's breathing becomes modified and restricted in various ways, not just momentarily, but habitually. We develop unhealthy habits without being aware of it. We tend to assume positions (slouched positions) that diminish lung capacities and take shortened breaths. We also live in social conditions that are not good for the health of our respiratory system.

Benefits of Deep Breathing

Improvement in the quality of the blood

This aids in the elimination of toxins from the system. Increase in the digestion and assimilation of food. The digestive organs such as the stomach receive more oxygen, and hence operate more efficiently. The digestion is further enhanced by the fact that the food is oxygenated more.

Improvement in the nervous system

This is due again to the increased oxygenation and hence nourishment of the nervous system. This improves the health of the whole body, since the nervous system communicates to all parts of the body.

Rejuvenation of pituitary and pineal glands

The brain has a special affinity for oxygen, requiring three times more oxygen than does the rest of the body. This has far-reaching effects on our well-being.

Rejuvenation of the skin

The skin becomes smoother and a reduction of facial wrinkles occurs.

The movements of the diaphragm

During the deep breathing exercise massage the abdominal organs - the stomach, small intestine, liver and pancreas. The upper movement of the diaphragm also massages the heart. This stimulates the blood circulation in these organs. The lungs become healthy and powerful, a good insurance against respiratory problems.

Deep, slow, yoga breathing reduces heart's workload

The result is a more efficient, stronger heart that operates better and lasts longer. It also mean reduced blood pressure and less heart disease. The yoga breathing exercises reduce the workload on the heart in two ways-

- Deep-breathing leads to more efficient lungs, which means more oxygen is brought into contact with blood sent to the lungs by the heart. So, the heart doesn't have to work as hard to deliver oxygen to the tissues.

- Deep breathing leads to a greater pressure differential in the lungs, which leads to an increase in the circulation, thus resting the heart a little. Deep, slow breathing assists in weight control. If you are overweight, the extra oxygen burns up the excess fat more efficiently. If you are underweight, the extra oxygen feeds the starving tissues and glands. In other words, yoga tends to produce the ideal weight for you.

Relaxation of the mind and body

Slow, deep, rhythmic breathing causes a reflex stimulation of the parasympathetic nervous system, which results in a reduction in the heart rate and relaxation of the muscles. These two factors cause a reflex relaxation of the mind, since the mind and body are very interdependent. In addition, oxygenation of the brain tends to normalise brain function, reducing excessive anxiety levels. The breathing exercises cause an increase in the elasticity of the lungs and rib cage. This creates an increased breathing capacity all day, not just during the actual exercise period. This means all the above benefits also occur all day.

Pranayama is a vital scientific and therapeutic aspect of yoga. It is the breathing process or the control of the motion of inhalation, exhalation and the retention of vital energy. By controlling Prana (life force), one can control all the forces of the universe, namely, gravity, magnetism, electricity and nerve currents.

During Pranayarna inhalation stimulates the system and fills the lungs with fresh air; retention raises the internal temperature and plays an important part in increasing the absorption of oxygen; and finally exhalation causes the diaphragm to return to the original position and air full of toxins and impurities is forced out by the contraction of inter-costal muscles.

These are the main components of Pranayama that massage the abdominal muscles and tone up the working of various organs of the body. Due to the proper functions of these organs, vital energy flows to all the systems. The success of Pranayama depends on proper ratio being maintained between inhalation, exhalation and retention.

■ ■